Drama Activities with Older Adults:

A Handbook for Leaders

Anne H. Thurman is Professor of Theater at Northwestern University and has been a national leader in the field of Creative Drama for many years. She has much firsthand experience leading drama sessions with seniors.

Carol Ann Piggins is Director of Creative Education Associates in Racine, Wisconsin and has extensive experience in the area of Creative Drama. She writes for many regional and national publications and is a frequent contributor to the *Instructor*.

Drama Activities with Older Adults:

A Handbook for Leaders

Anne H. Thurman
Carol Ann Piggins

Activities, Adaptation & Aging
Volume 2, Numbers 2/3

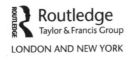

Routledge
Taylor & Francis Group

LONDON AND NEW YORK

Transferred to Digital Printing 2008 by Routledge
270 Madison Ave, New York NY 10016
2 Park Square, Milton Park, Abingdon, Oxon, OX14 4RN

First Published by

The Haworth Press, Inc., 10 Alice Street, Binghamton, NY 13904-1580

Paperback edition published in 1996.

Library of Congress Cataloging-in-Publication Data

Thurman, Anne.
    Drama activities with older adults.

    (Activities, adaptation & aging : v. 2., no 2/3)
    Bibliography: p.
    Includes index.
    1. Drama–Therapeutic use. 2. Aged–Mental health. 3. Nursing homes–Recreational activi-
ties. I. Piggins, Carol Ann. II. Title. III. Series.
RC952.5.A24 vol. 2, no. 2/3   362'.05s   82-11861
[RC451.4.A5]   [615.8'515]
ISBN 0-86656-167-6
ISBN 0-7890-6037-X (pbk)

Publisher's Note
The publisher has gone to great lengths to ensure the quality
of this reprint but points out that some imperfections in the original may be apparent.

Drama Activities with Older Adults:
A Handbook for Leaders

Activities, Adaptation & Aging
Volume 2, Numbers 2/3

Contents

FOREWORD

During the past ten years, I have had the opportunity, as a high school Drama teacher, to do a great deal of work with Theatre Games, Improvisation and Creative Dramatics. The context of my work has always been educational and child-centered, and, until recently, I had never seriously considered the idea of using Drama with older adults. Despite a background that included being raised in a household in which activities for Seniors was a frequent topic of conversation, I simply did not make the now obvious connection between senior citizens and Drama.

In 1980, I embarked on a MA degree program through the Educational Theatre Department of New York University. It began with a summer of study at Bretton Hall College of the Arts in Yorkshire England. That summer, I began to develop an awareness of the nearly limitless number of uses of drama activities. The many fine teachers and practitioners of drama that I encountered that summer had worked with all ages and types of people, using drama to entertain, but also to teach and to enlighten. At that time I became aware of the efficacy of drama as a tool for self-awareness. As a teacher, however, my consciousness was still focused on children; I had not yet made the connection between Drama and older adults.

In 1982, Phyllis Foster, editor of *Activities, Adaptation & Aging* (and not coincidentally, my mother), asked me if I would like to look at a manuscript that was to become this double issue of the journal. I willingly perused the manuscript with her, and what I found was an honest-to-God handbook for using Drama Activities with Older Adults. As I delved into the material, herewith presented, I was once more reminded of the universality of Drama and its applicability to all groups and all ages.

What you are about to read is, quite literally, a handbook. This is not a dusty monument of a book to be filed on a shelf somewhere. This is a working book. If you work with Drama and older adults, this is your guide, and it should be always in your hands, the pages dog-eared, notes written in the margins, key ideas underlined and particularly exciting thoughts circled. In a very short time, you will find it your constant companion and true friend as a book really ought to be.

It will also be a stepping-stone however, because doing drama is doing creative work. As you work with the exercises in this book you will find your own creativity challenged as new ideas come to you. Put these new ideas to work as well, so that the handbook becomes not only your foundation for doing drama but also the impetus to carry the activities even further. Use the handbook as a guide; ultimately, through practice, you will develop your own techniques and methods of working, inspired by your use of this book.

Finally, since many of you using this book will be new to the field, a word of warning about Drama is necessary. It is a very risky business. Those of you who are highly concerned with "results" will find it necessary to relax a bit, because with each group, some things will work and some will not. Today's hit is tomorrow's flop, or at least has that potential. Don't be distressed if you run into snags; regroup and try again using a different approach, a different slant on the material, or even abandon and start anew. All of these courses of action are acceptable for the practitioners of Drama. You will have great successes as well which are also part of the risk-taking process and hence part of Drama. Finally, Drama is Life; what could be more appropriate for use with older adults? Enjoy yourselves.

Kenneth J. Foster
Littleton, Colorado
1982

PREFACE

This book is addressed to activity directors, recreation specialists, social workers, psychiatric nurses, occupational and other therapists as well as administrators and volunteers who work with older adults. The materials presented here are of a practical nature and are applicable to the populations found in nursing and retirement homes, day care and community centers.

The need of older persons for adequate food, clothing, shelter and medical care is widely acknowledged in our country, although the means for meeting these needs is not agreed upon. Only recently have the emotional and psychological needs of people age 65 and older been given the recognition they deserve. Those who work with seniors in residential homes and community centers are aware of the devastating effects of the losses experienced by our elderly population—loss of job, spouse, friends, independence, hearing and/or eyesight. Professionals and volunteers in the field of geriatrics are challenged daily by the effects of these losses—isolation, depression, dependence, hopelessness. If the walls can be breached and the barriers overcome, the riches of an entire lifetime can be revealed and valued.

Looking upon growing older in more positive terms convinced us to adapt the philosophy and methods of creative drama for use with older adults. We believed creative drama could bring forth their unrealized potential for creativity. We felt it could reestablish communication skills, allow for ventilation of hostile and negative feelings, and provide the status and recognition so desperately needed by many seniors. We knew that creative drama, being a social art, could mitigate against feelings of depression and isolation. Calling for physical as well as verbal expression of ideas, thoughts and feelings, creative drama could encourage freedom of movement from bodies that have become inert and voices that have become stilled. Since creative drama depends on spontaneous, not scripted interchange, it could keep participants in the present, the now, but allow them to draw on all the memories of the past. We felt this kind of drama could overcome a sense of powerlessness and dependency since it places the player in the center of decision making and could bring about a shift from preoccupation with self and physical needs to a concern for needs of the group. Since it depends on the imagination, creative drama could lead seniors to consider what might be as well as what is. Our experience has shown us that our assumptions were correct. Creative drama is an effective tool for meeting the psychological and emotional needs of older adults.

All of the activities described in the book have been tested with groups of seniors. Much of the material in the book has grown out of workshops with activity directors and other professionals who work with older adults. These workshops of eight sessions each were held in 1978, 1979, and 1980. They were sponsored by the North Light Repertory Theatre in Evanston, Illinois as part of their community outreach program. Funds for the workshop were provided by the McCormick Charitable Trust of Chicago, which has a special interest in meeting the needs of the elderly. Most of the workshop participants were professionals actively working in homes and centers at the time, but only a very few had previous training or experience with drama. The workshop program provided a variety of learning experiences aimed at developing leadership skills. These experiences included pre-drama games and exercises designed to overcome fears and develop trust and a sense of community; improvisations to develop verbal fluency and spontaneity; role playing to increase empathy and develop an understanding of diverse characters; and story dramatization to apprehend dramatic form. In addition, workshop participants observed demonstrations of creative drama either on videotape or live in a home or center. Some time was spent in small group work which allowed participants to practice leading one another in drama exercises. A good deal of time was spent in discussion and evaluation of all the above activities. A one-half hour videotape has been edited showing the work of two workshop participants and is available for in-service training and professional meetings.

The role of the activity director, nurse, therapist, recreation specialist is a crucial link between the older adults and all that they have experienced with all that they can become. The quality and variety of a recreational program in a center or home, then, depends on the imagination, skills and confidence of the leader. Few training programs provide a background in all of the recreational areas that are required to meet the needs of the senior population. This book attempts to give the leader the background and skills necessary to lead a creative drama group. Along with a discussion of the value of drama for older adults, there are games, exercises, and fully developed drama session plans encompassing areas such as sensory awareness, imagination, movement and pantomime, improvisation and story dramatization.

We believe that every person is born with the capacity to not only take in impressions of the world, but also to express a reaction to all that he has taken in and finally to transform those impressions and reactions into some unique statement. If no one shows an interest in those expressions, they may go underground or they may become lost, depriving the individual of his connectedness with the world. The reaction/activity director who makes use of his or her own creative powers and who uses the dramatic mode to unleash the imagination of the elderly to activate memories, to revive the spirit of play and to channel the emotions of the group will be richly rewarded personally and will do much to reaffirm the positive life force of older adults.

A. H. Thurman
C. A. Piggins

ACKNOWLEDGMENTS

Drama Activities with Older Adults is a result of assistance and support from many people and organizations. We wish to thank the following:

*Gregory Kandell, founder and first director of the North Light Repertory Theatre, Evanston, Illinois, for initiating a program at the Levy Senior Center and sponsoring the three years of workshops.

*McCormick Charitable Trust for their generous and continuing funding of the workshops which allowed seventy-five professionals to receive training in drama leadership.

*Lisa Wilson and Mary Monroe who handled the publicity, brochures and other administrative details from the North Light Theatre.

*Mary Christel who assisted so efficiently during the first year's workshop.

*Dawn Murray for her penetrating photographs and valuable manuscript assistance.

*Lynn Gartley for directing and editing of the videotape.

*Marilyn Richman and Mollie Grabeman for their skillful demonstrations in two different homes for seniors.

*The readers of the pilot handbook who gave greatly valued suggestions for the revision: Phyllis Foster, Marilyn Lamken, Patricia Sawyer, Geraldine B. Siks, Nadia Weisberg.

*Workshop participants from the years 1978 and 1979 who taught us much and convinced us of the need of the present publication.

*Workshop participants from the year 1980 who read and evaluated the pilot manuscript.

*Nancy Yeoh who first interested one of the authors in the tremendous possibilities of drama for seniors, and to Natalia Deutsch who, with the Evanston Mental Health Society, sponsored a workshop in 1973.

*Judi Schuetze and Deborah Blaustein for their patience with the authors and painstaking typing of the manuscript.

Chapter 1

INTRODUCING CREATIVE DRAMA

A Tale of Two Women

Mary Sullivan lives in a nursing home. She sits in her room—alone. Perhaps once a month her niece visits her for an hour or so. But otherwise Mrs. Sullivan sits alone. The TV, purchased by her son before he moved out of state, is often turned on, but Mrs. Sullivan doesn't watch it. She stares. She stares at the floor. She stares at nothing.

Eighty now, Mrs. Sullivan feels that her life is over, she is waiting to die. She speaks in monosyllables if at all. She rarely smiles. She eats little and refuses to participate in any of the craft or social activities the activity director has planned. In some ways Mary is lucky. Fifty percent of nursing home residents have no living relative or no direct relationship with one.[1] At least she sees her niece once a month and hears from her son by telephone occasionally. But most of the time Mrs. Sullivan sits in her room alone. Doing nothing.

Jean Terry lives in the same nursing home. She too is eighty, but Mrs. Terry is quite busy. It's not that she has more company. She never had children, her husband died years ago, and she has few living relatives. But Mrs. Terry participates in many of the home's activities. She belongs to a card club. She plays bingo. She does volunteer work for the Red Cross and on Thursdays she goes to drama club.

"I used to sit around feeling sorry for myself," she confides, "but then our activity director started this creative drama group." Of course Mrs. Jensen, the activity director, didn't call it drama at first. She invited residents to an auction. The invitation said money would be provided and not many could refuse an offer like that. "I remember," Jean Terry continues, "that I didn't feel just right that day. My joints ached and I was tired, but I was so curious about what Mrs. Jensen was up to that I went.

"We had such a good time. We had a thousand dollars worth of play money and Mr. Gibbs, the business manager, auctioned off the most outlandish things—a garter worn by Gypsy Rose Lee, a ruffled lamp shade owned by Marie Antoinette! I won a set of wooden false teeth used by George Washington. They still sit on my book shelf."

When Mrs. Jensen suggested that the group meet every Thursday to create other scenarios, Jean couldn't resist. She became a regular.

"As the weeks went by we had a lot more fun. We were involved in movement exercises, stretching as though getting up in the morning, or growing like flowers, or pretending we were prospecting for gold in the Colorado Rockies. Never thought anyone would catch me doing some of those silly things—but they were fun and for some reason, I wasn't having so many aches and pains!

"And we made up scenes. One time we talked about all the things we did in high school. We chose some of them to dramatize. They gave me something else to think about, for I had a part to play.

"I got to know some of the other residents better. Mrs. Kelly invited me to join the card club and I did. I was never much for cards, but I liked being with Mrs. Kelly and the others. Well, one thing led to another and pretty soon I found myself playing bingo on Mondays and helping out by stuffing envelopes for the Red Cross on Fridays. I'm so busy now, I hardly have time to feel sorry for myself. Guess I'm going to have to live another ten years to get everything done I want to get done!"

The Nature of Creative Drama

What is this creative drama that made such a difference in Mrs. Terry's life?

Creative drama is the improvisational, non-exhibitional form of drama in which participants are led to imagine, enact and reflect upon human experience.[2] Whereas the performers in traditional theatre depend upon a script, the participants in creative drama use no script. Rather their drama is improvised from their own life experiences or situations suggested by the leader or themselves, eventually. Participants use their imaginations to develop spontaneous dialogue and accompanying movement to take on a role in the drama they evolve with the leader.

They share this experience for their own enjoyment and re-creation rather than for performance. They do it for each other, *not* an audience. Through the drama and the discussion following it they explore what it means to be human. Their recreation truly becomes a means of re-creation.

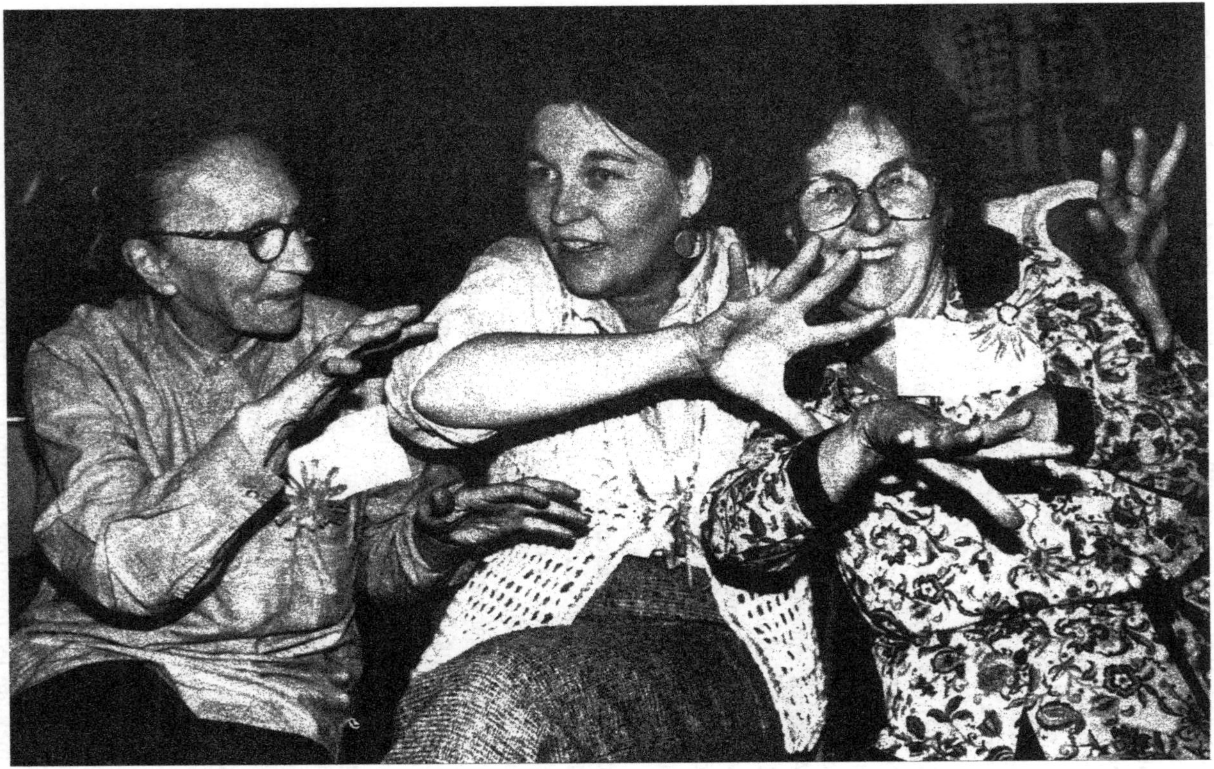

Photo by Dawn Murray

Verbal games, pantomime, creative movement, role playing, improvisation and play making are all aspects of creative drama. In a verbal game, players are challenged to think quickly and to concentrate. In pantomime, specific activities, like baking a cake, are carried out with appropriate movements but no words. Creative movement can get players involved in reacting to a color, a rhythm or music using only hands and arms or using the entire body.

In role playing players take on the persona of someone else. They become a tyrannical employer, a timid salesman or a swashbuckling pirate with the license to experience ways of behavior very different from their own. Working in pairs or small groups participants take on roles to explore relationships and attitudes: Role playing activities are relatively free in form with no clearly defined beginning, middle or end and no specific problems to be solved.

Although improvisation uses role playing, it goes a step beyond in that a given set of circumstances is provided, including a problem to be solved. In their roles, players work through the problems toward some kind of resolution. Dialogue is spontaneous and solutions may vary from group to group. For example, players, working in pairs, might be given the following motivation: "You are all in a mountain valley panning for gold. Suddenly you discover what you're looking for. Unfortunately, in each pair, both of you lay claim to the same site. What will happen?" Each pair, working at the same time, may come up with very different solutions. One scene may end in a shout out, another may involve a complicated legal battle, still another may end in compromise.

Play making uses many of the same elements as improvisation. The dialogue is still spontaneous, but more group planning is involved and more consideration given to how the drama might look. The structure is frequently provided by a narrative poem, short story, newspaper feature or historical event. Such material can give a strong plot line, with action that grows out of the conflict, well delineated characters and a satisfying ending. A modest work of art is being created.

Whereas theatre makes use of scenery, costumes, lighting and makeup to create an illusion, creative drama calls upon the participants to imagine the darkness of the cave, the warmth of the fire, the ill-fitting clothes and the mud streaked faces. Participants use their imagination to create belief in the dramatic situation. In all facets of creative drama participants are led to use their imaginations. In addition, their skills of concentration, observation, problem solving and communication are sharpened and they are led to explore emotions and attitudes.

Values of Creative Drama to Older Adults

We know that a large number of the elderly face difficult problems. Many feel isolated, they live alone with few visitors and diminishing power over their lives. There is often loneliness and accompanying depression. For many older adults, boredom is a constant companion. There seems to be no energy and no will to participate in life or what it has to offer. Fear of crime and insufficient finances present very real problems for many senior citizens as do fears of failing health, loss of sensory function and other manifestations of aging. Still others experience lowered self esteem and feelings of unimportance or uselessness.

Although drama cannot solve all these problems, it can at least provide a forum for exploring attitudes towards them. The simple fact of being together in a drama group, which encourages interaction, helps alleviate feelings of isolation, loneliness and depression. Participants learn that they are not alone, that other people share many of the same fears, complaints and problems. A drama group legitimizes their feelings. Human contact can help to reawaken feelings of involvement, of caring. Drama helps provide meaning again.

Participants who have been repressing hostility, fear or frustration can find release by stepping into someone else's shoes. Mrs. Barker may be feeling fearful of moving into a retirement home, a move being forced on her by her children. Through playing the role of a teenager who is being forced to go to college against her will, she may be able to work through some of her own feelings. Mrs. Barker may be able to vent some of her hostility and release some of the anger she feels about losing control over her own life.

Mr. Geminaro constantly interrupts other seniors at the community center. He insists on dominating every conversation. By casting him in the role of a master carpenter who is explaining the best way to pound a nail to a new apprentice, and instructing the apprentice to play the role of a student who gets everything mixed up and who continually interrupts his teacher, a leader can help Mr. Geminaro confront his behavior. Through discussion after the role playing, Mr. Geminaro can be led to discover for himself what it feels like to be interrupted. That insight may help him change his behavior.

Many elderly find themselves living more and more in the past. As they near the end of their life, a summing up, a kind of ongoing mental review of feelings, experience and relationships occurs. Remembering what one did can help validate one's existence. "I lived. I was here. I did these things. I made a difference." When much of one's life is past, it is not surprising that one looks back. But drama can help to anchor that backward look firmly in the present. It values memories, using them as the raw material for art. A drama group provides the opportunity for continuity at a time when many seniors have experienced a great deal of discontinuity. They may have lost jobs, spouses or homes. Long established lines have been broken. Creative drama can provide the opportunity to find linkage between what was once and what is now.

The elderly have a need to love and to be loved, to feel secure emotionally. They need to relax, to have fun, to laugh. They need to belong to and retain a role of importance in the society in which they live. They need to explore new ways to play a meaningful role. They need to be productive and to receive recognition for their accomplishments and efforts. They need to have a voice and a choice in the way their lives are lived and to retain their feelings of dignity and self respect.

Drama can provide a forum for meeting these basic human needs. Because creative drama is process oriented, it, by its very nature, demands participation, involvement, commitment. Group members have a great deal of input in determining what will happen, and often a feeling of pride in working together to create a drama. Each person counts and a sense of belonging is gained as the group meets regularly over time.

Because divergent thought is rewarded far more than convergent thought, because creative drama is improvisational, springing from the raw material of life, everyone can feel a sense of accomplishment. There are many opportunities to gain recognition and praise because there are unlimited possibilities for meaningful and successful participation.

As seniors work together in drama, they have ever increasing opportunities for making choices. "Which warm up exercises should we use today? What characters will we need to dramatize the 'Secret Life of Walter Mitty?' What other daydreams might Walter Mitty have? How could we replay this scene to make it more interesting?" Having the forum for exercising their decision making powers in drama, participants may well take more interest in making choices in other areas of their lives.

We all know how much better we feel when there is something to look forward to. How much more energy we have. How much more interested in life we are. Participation in a creative drama group may just provide the spark some seniors need to rekindle their zest for life. The shared experience of an imaginative verbal game often produces much merriment and when people laugh together, when people have a

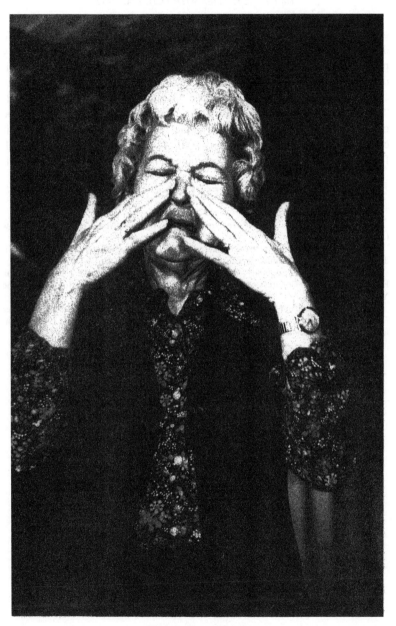

Photo by Dawn Murray

good time together, a camaraderie evolves. Again and again creative drama groups engender, through the enjoyable shared experiences they provide, a sense of caring. When there is joy in one part of our lives, it often lightens our entire existence.

The Report of the White House Conference on Aging says that, ". . . an individual has a right to *live* until he dies . . . the objective of rehabilitation should be the dynamic restoration to the fullest physical, mental and social productivity."[3] If we agree with that goal we will find the use of creative drama with older adults to be a most useful tool.

REFERENCES

1. Robert N. Butler, *Why Survive? Being Old in America.* New York: Harper & Row (1975) p. 210.

2. Jed H. Davis and Tom Behm. "Terminology of Drama/Theatre with and for Children: A Redefinition." Children's Theatre Review. Vol. XXVII, No. 1 (1978) 10-11.

This definition was originally developed by Anne Thurman, Ann M. Shaw and Frank Harland for the 1972 Congress of the International Association of Theatres for Children and Young People.

3. U. S. Department of Health, Education and Welfare. *The Nation and Its Older People: A Report of the White House Conference on Aging, January 9-12, 1961.* Washington, D.C.: Government Printing Office, April 1961.

Chapter 2

GETTING STARTED

Forming the Group

You've read about creative drama, or you've heard about it, or you've seen somebody else leading a creative drama group. You've given it some thought and you've decided that you want to form your own group, but you are apprehensive about how to begin. How, you wonder, do you get a group together?

Getting People Together

You may be able to piggyback your program with an already existing program to start with. You might initiate some creative movement during exercise time. Or you might play some inviting drama games during the intermission of the bingo club. After you've acquainted residents with your activity you could invite them to join you at a specified time in the future for more of the same in the new drama club.

Another way to piggyback is to invite an already existing drama group, either a senior group or a group from a local high school, college or community theatre to make a presentation at your facility. Later a time might be announced when your guests would return to lead a workshop with residents, thus establishing the drama group.

Of course, you may choose to take the direct approach and simply invite your residents or community center regulars to attend the first meeting of a new drama club. Other staff members could be enlisted to help drum up enthusiasm. You can create further interest by sending written invitations, distributing fliers or printing an announcement in your newsletter. Inviting people to attend in person or over the phone also gives you an opportunity to explain your program.

On the other hand, if you think the people you work with would resist participating in a drama club, either because they are afraid they do not have enough "talent" or because anything new frightens them, you may want to use an indirect approach. Instead of calling the first meeting "drama" call it something else, something exciting, something familiar, something enticing. Residents may, for example, be invited to an auction (see p. 123), to the mock trial of a popular staff member for some outlandish "crime," or to the "filming of a TV program" like "What's My Life?," "Queen for a Day," or "Dialing for Dollars." Perhaps an interesting, famous person (played by another staff member) is to visit the facility and everyone is invited to meet him or her and get autographs. Possibilities are Elizabeth Taylor, Hank Aaron, Bob Hope, Phyllis Diller, Mahalia Jackson or Prince Charles and Lady Diana.

Another gambit is to plan a "This is Your Life" tribute for a resident or staff member. Everyone else can be in on the secret and can help plan the surprise. Or a treasure hunt could be planned. All "hunters" could have safari hats and clues that are imaginative and fun. After residents participate and find that they have a good time, they can be invited to form a creative drama group which will continue to provide similar good times.

Formalizing the Group

Before beginning, you need to think some things through. How large will your group be? If you'll have help you may be able to handle twelve or fifteen. If you're leading the group by yourself you may only want eight or ten.

What room will you use? Will there be enough space for movement activities? Is the room well ventilated? Will the room be warm enough in winter and cool enough in the summer for the comfort of participants? Above all you will want to avoid rooms that are used as thoroughfares or that are particularly noisy.

How long do you want your sessions to be? Half an hour is probably not long enough to get anything going. More than an hour will be too tiring.

At the first session it will be important to set the tone. You will want to use the name of each participant and be sure to make some personal comment to each. A hand shake or other physical contact is important as well. Especially at the beginning, it is helpful to have the group sitting in a circle. Everyone can then see well and everyone shares the same status, one of importance.

At first, you will want to use unison activities in which everyone participates at the same time. This not only keeps everyone interested, but it also eliminates feelings of tension or fear of failure because no one has to "perform" in front of anyone else. The leader should stress that the drama will be improvisational. There will be no script and no memorization of lines.

A unifying theme such as an auction (see Chapter 6) rather than a string of unrelated activities helps to make the session more meaningful. Within the unified theme, it is important to vary the type of activity so that some are more, some are less active. A change of tempo helps to maintain interest and avoids overtiring participants.

Discovering Individual Abilities/Interests

It is important to provide time, especially in early sessions, to discuss feelings, to talk about ourselves, to get to know each other. This will also give the leader an opportunity to find out about the abilities, talents and interests of group members. Perhaps one member knows a lot about photography and would love to serve as "official" photographer. Perhaps another plays the piano and yet another the guitar. Several may sing well and there may be dancers too. Information about hobbies, occupation and travel may be shared as well. Whatever the interests and abilities, they can become an invaluable part of the drama. It may be helpful to have participants fill out an interests inventory.

Perhaps most important of all in assuring that participants will return is the attitude and ability of the leader. Leadership skills are discussed in Chapter 4. If you are enthusiastic, sensitive and caring everyone will feel welcome. If you demonstrate a good sense of humor, if you invite participation, if you ask questions and really listen to the answers, seniors are bound to want to come back to your group. If you make your drama group irresistible, there won't be many who stay away. You'll be on your way.

Breaking the Ice

Although seniors may live in the same retirement or nursing home or attend the same community center they may not be well acquainted or even know each other's names. Some are shut out by the formation of cliques, others shut themselves out. How to break the ice becomes a real challenge as the leader starts a drama group.

This section suggests a number of pre-drama games and activities in-

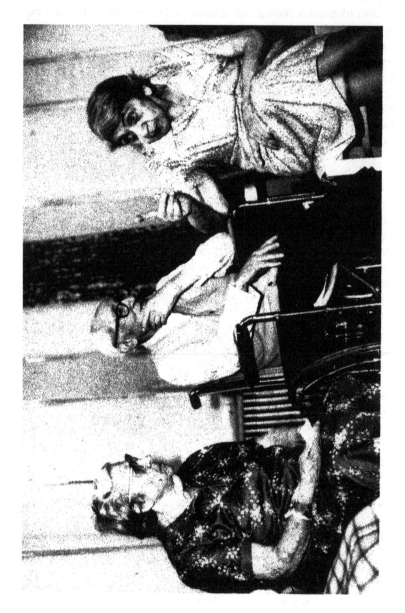

tended to help participants get acquainted and feel comfortable with each other. Activities like "Copy Cat" requiring the group to move and/or speak simultaneously help establish a climate of low threat and high enjoyment. Games like "Information Please" provide the security of a circle, within which seniors can exchange life experiences and explore likenesses and differences. Games such as "Pass It On" help to develop group spirit and cohesion in addition to meeting the need for physical closeness and warmth.

These activities help seniors concentrate, increase their attention span, trust their own ideas, share their feelings sincerely, participate with greater alertness and energy and enjoy interacting with others. They can be used as warm ups in a newly formed drama group or as activities to piggyback with some other programming.

The objectives given for each activity indicate the desired behavior for participants. Each activity may well accomplish many things other than those indicated, of course, but only a few key objectives have been selected for each. This will allow for focus and quick assessment of whether or not the exercise was successful.

"Information Please," for example, is played to help participants learn each other's names and share background information. At the same time it allows each participant an opportunity to make a contribution to the group and to speak out loud in a group situation. The leader's concern at the beginning, though, is getting people to feel comfortable with each other, and learning each other's names is an important step toward that goal. As you play the game, it is an easy matter to determine if your objectives are being met. You have your objectives clearly in mind. From time to time you may wish to list objectives for yourself as leader in addition to those indicated for the group.

Following the objectives, you will find detailed directions for playing the game or carrying out the activity. Any phrases to be spoken by the leader are indicated in italic print.

For several of the activities, further developments or variations are also indicated. Once players are comfortable with a drama game or exercise, you may wish to make it a bit more challenging or interesting. In "Information Please," for example, once players have learned the playing pattern and are quite comfortable tossing the ball to one another and repeating each other's names, you may wish to develop the activity by asking additional information about hobbies, birthplace, funny incidents, favorite radio program before TV, etc.

Necessary materials are indicated for each pre-drama game or activity following the directions, development or variation.

Activities appear in order of ascending difficulty. "Information Please," for example, is a very simple, though enjoyable activity. "Categories" is more difficult and "This Is a Pen" is more difficult yet. It is important to start with simpler activities first, building the confidence of the group before moving to more difficult ones. It is also important not to play any of these pre-drama games or activities too long. Ten or fifteen minutes of enjoyable play is far preferable to half an hour of tedium.

INFORMATION PLEASE

Objectives: Learn each other's names, share background information.

Share background information: hobbies, occupations, preferences.

Develop an atmosphere of acceptance, comfort and trust.

Directions: Sit or stand in a circle.

Leader says, *My name is . . . , what's yours?* Leader looks directly at the person questioned and throws a bean bag or ball to that person. The second person repeats, *My name is . . . what's yours?* and throws the bean bag to a third person. Continue the activity until all have introduced themselves.

Development: Additional areas of information might include:

1. *My hobby is . . . , what's yours?*
2. *I was born in . . . , where were you born?*
3. *The first car I rode in was a . . .*
4. *My family moved . . . times by the time I was twenty.*
5. *The worst accident I can remember in our town/ city was . . .*
6. *The funniest thing that ever happened in my family was . . .*
7. *Before TV my favorite radio program was . . .*

Materials: bean bag or large, plastic beach ball

Note: The ball helps the group focus attention on the speaker. Receiving and holding the ball is a gentle press for participation. When players feel more comfortable, information may be shared around the circle without using a bean bag or ball.

HOW DO YOU FEEL ABOUT?

Objectives: Develop spontaneity and confidence in expressing feelings, values and attitudes.
Accept and value feelings and attitudes different from one's own.

Directions: Sit or stand in a circle.

Leader says, *I hate . . . (spinach, pollution, football). What do you hate, Betty?* Betty responds and repeats the question to another person in the circle. Continue until all or many have had the opportunity to respond. To help group focus on the speaker, the leader may toss a bean bag or a ball as he or she says, *What is your pet peeve, Mary?*

Development: Other types of feelings and attitudes might include:
My pet peeve is . . .
My fondest dream is . . .
When I'm angry, I . . .
I really like . . .
The nicest thing about a friend is . . .
As a child I was most afraid of . . .
If I had a thousand dollars, I'd . . .
My biggest disappointment in high school was . . .
The thing that makes me happiest is . . .

Materials: Bean bag, beach ball, or Nerf ball (optional)

COPY CAT

Objectives: Sharpen ability to observe.

Move rhythmically and in unison with others.

Adapt quickly to changes in movement and tempo.

Overcome fear of participation.

Directions: Sit or stand in a circle.

Choose one player as "IT" who must leave the room.

Choose a leader who must start a simple action which can be easily repeated (scratching head, patting shoulder, clapping hands, etc.).

The group must imitate and continue the action of the leader. "IT" returns to the room, stands in the center of the circle observing the actions of the group.

The leader attempts to change actions as often as possible without being caught by "IT." The group must follow the change of actions without giving away the identity of the leader.

"IT" has three guesses to establish the identity of the leader.

Materials: None

PASS IT ON

Objectives: Develop feeling of belonging and relate to others physically.

Reproduce volume, tone quality, pitch, inflection and/or gesture of previous player.

Directions: Sit or stand in a circle. The leader directs a phrase, sound or action to the person on his or her right. For example, the leader might make a funny face. The receiver of the action makes a similar face to the person on his or her right. This continues until all have received and passed on the original action. Sounds or phrases can also be passed on. If the group is comfortable together, hand shakes, hugs, etc. may be passed.

Development:	Possible words or phrases:	*Hello*
		I like you
		You're great
		My friend
	Possible sounds:	sh-h-h
		bz-z-z
		hum
	Possible actions:	smile/frown
		yawn
		pat on hand
		hand shake/squeeze
		hug
		kiss on cheek

Variation: When passing on words or phrases, ask each person to use a different inflection or voice quality.

Materials: None

Note: This game should be played at a brisk pace for maximum effectiveness. As the speed picks up, the energy level of the whole group raises. Because some individuals may be somewhat reluctant to touch, touch responses have been placed last on the list.

CATEGORIES

Objectives: Increased mental alertness through active listening and association of ideas.
Develop flexibility in thinking.

Directions: Group sits or stands in a circle with "IT" standing in the center. As "IT" slowly pivots he or she extends one arm outward. Upon stopping and pointing to one person in the circle, he or she calls out one of the following categories: *Earth, Air, Fire, Water.* The person pointed at must respond as follows:

> *Earth* = the name of an animal living on the earth
> *Air* = the name of a bird/animal that moves through sky
> *Water* = the name of an animal that lives in the water
> *Fire* = one word: "Help" (loudly)

"IT" pivots again, stops, points to another person, calls out another category and so on. After several exchanges, a new player may be "IT." Once an animal has been named it should not be repeated. Instead of pointing, "IT" can throw a bean bag or ball to the person who is to respond next.

Variation: Instead of using the single word "Help" in response to "Fire," the group can be challenged to make various free associations with Fire, such as:

Sun spots	Forest fires
Flames	Wiener roast
"Ouch"	Mrs. O'Leary
Fire truck	

Materials: None

CLAP, SNAP, NAME GAME

Objectives: Learn names.
Increase concentration, attention and listening.

Directions: Form a circle. Leader demonstrates the rhythmic sequence of the game by saying the words in the chant and simultaneously doing the actions that accompany them.

WORDS	ACTIONS
1. *pat*	pat thighs with palm of hand
2. *pat*	" "
3. *clap*	clap hands
4. *clap*	" "
5. *snap*	snap fingers
6. *snap*	" "

Repeat this much of the game with the group saying and doing the words and actions. This short sequence may need to be repeated several times until the words and actions are coordinated.

Now, names of group members will be substituted in steps 5 and 6. The leader begins saying first his or her name and next the name of another player who then becomes "IT." The complete sequence will look like this:

WORDS	ACTIONS
1. *pat*	pat thighs with palm of hand
2. *pat*	" "
3. *clap*	clap hands
4. *clap*	" "
5. *Gene*	snap fingers
6. *Mary*	" "

The leader should establish and maintain a tempo slow enough so that the group can keep the rhythm without a break. As the group becomes more familiar with the names and more responsive to the rhythm, the tempo may be increased. When the group becomes very adept at the game, they can do actions only on steps 1-4 omitting the words.

Materials: None

Note: For those who find clapping and snapping difficult or painful, a stick or cane to hit the floor and/or a maraca could be substituted.

THIS IS A PEN

Objectives: Develop mental alertness and quickness of response. Work together to maintain rhythm.

Directions: Sit or stand in a circle.

Leader explains and demonstrates the following sequence:

Leader:	*This is a pen* (hands to person to the right, person 1)
Person 1:	*A what?* (takes pen)
Leader:	*A pen*
Person 1:	*Oh, a pen*

*　　*　　*

Person 1:	*This is a pen* (gives pen to person to the right, person 2)
Person 2:	*A what?* (takes pen)
Person 1:	*A what?* (turns to leader)
Leader:	*A pen.*
Person 1:	*A pen.* (turns to person 2)
Person 2:	*Oh, a pen.*

*　　*　　*

Person 2:	*This is a pen* (hands a pen to person to the right, person 3)
Person 3:	*A. what?* (takes pen)
Person 2:	*A what?* (turns to person 1)

> *Person 1:*   A *what?* (turns to leader)
> *Leader:*   A *pen*
> *Person 1:*   A *pen* (to person 2)
> *Person 2:*   A *pen* (to person 3)
> *Person 3:*   Oh, *a pen*

Try the above very slowly until the pattern and rhythm are established. Then start again from the beginning and allow speed to build as play moves all around the circle.

Materials: A pen or a cup, book or any object with a one syllable name.

PICTURE CHARADES

Objectives: Work together to solve a problem.
Communicate non-verbally.

Directions: Form groups of 5-6. Each group should be seated close together on the floor or at a table. Give each group felt tip pens and drawing paper. After explaining the game, the leader asks each group to send a representative to the center of the room. The leader tells and/or shows them the name of one animal. The representative must rush back to their own group and begin drawing the given animal. The "artist" must not give any pantomimic or verbal hints except to answer *yes* or *no* as the group tries to guess the animal. The first group to guess correctly is the winner. Ask players to guess quietly so that one group does not overhear the correct answer from another. Give players enough time to try to discover the answer on their own.

After groups have guessed the first animal, repeat the procedure with new artists from each group. Continue until each person has had a chance to draw for his or her group.

Development: Possible animals to draw and guess:

octopus	zebra	elephant
mouse	rabbit	ant
snake	alligator	butterfly
camel	dachshund	centipede
whale	beaver	turtle
lion	swordfish	kangaroo
moose	dragon	

Another category is Famous Monuments/Landmarks:

Eiffel Tower	Old Faithful
Washington Monument	Niagara Falls
Golden Gate Bridge	Mt. Rushmore
St. Louis Arch	Leaning Tower of Pisa
Any local landmarks	

Other possible categories:

Disasters	Machines
Foods	Trees/flowers

Variation: For non-ambulatory groups, the leader can go around to each group and whisper what is to be drawn to the person whose turn it is to be artist. To ensure fairness, these people should not begin drawing until leader gives a signal so all start at the same time.

Materials: Felt tip pens (at least one per group), 8½ x 11 sheets of paper, 5 x 7 cards with the name of an animal on each.

Chapter 3

IN THE BEGINNING

In early sessions participants may be reluctant to become involved. The concept of creative drama may be new to them and they may resist risking involvement until they have had an opportunity to size up the situation. It is often the leader's willingness to "play," the leader's pleasure in taking on a role, that gradually wins first cooperation and then enthusiastic participation.

In Chapter 6, planning an entire drama session around a single theme will be discussed. In the early sessions, however, the leader, and participants, may feel more comfortable doing shorter, more self-contained exercises or activities. Whether the leader chooses an activity that helps to awaken the senses, to stimulate movement or to stretch the imagination, he or she can use it to challenge participants and get the ball rolling in drama.

This chapter is divided into two parts. The first introduces some frequently used creative drama techniques that will be helpful in leading the activities that follow. The second describes activities to stimulate the senses and heighten powers of observation and concentration, activities for movement and activities for exercising the imagination. Participant objectives are indicated for each activity and directions are given in detail. Those activities suggested first in each category are easiest to carry out and least threatening to participants. As the confidence level of the leader and participants increases, more difficult activities can be tried.

Important Creative Drama Techniques

Simultaneous Play. All participants are moving and/or speaking at the same time. For example, the leader might ask players to imagine that the room is a circus and then direct them to imagine that they are all jugglers. At a given signal all will pantomime juggling balls, then pins, then lighted torches. Participants can engage in this activity while seated or standing. Next the leader will ask participants to imagine they are barkers at a side show. At a given signal, all the barkers will begin announcing their amazing attractions at the same time. One might be extolling the glories of the strong man, while another cries out for circus goers to come see the snake lady. This technique allows for experimentation at the same time that it provides a fairly tension free environment. Because everyone is participating at the same time there is protection through anonymity. No one is on the spot or being examined.

Warm Ups. Warm up activities are often used at the beginning of a session to break the ice and get people in the mood for relaxed spontaneous participation. Ideally the warm up is tied into the theme of the session. If the session has a picnic theme, for example, the warm up may be *Information Please*, using questions like, "What is your favorite place for a picnic?" or "What is the funniest thing that ever happened to you when you were on a picnic?" (See "Breaking the Ice" in Chapter 2).

Freezing. When the leader calls out the signal "freeze," all players instantly stop whatever they are doing and momentarily hold the position they were in when the signal was given. This allows the leader to give the next instruction, comment on the activity or discuss another point with participants. The shake of a tambourine or clapping of hands works well as a signal.

Side Coaching. While players are doing a pantomime activity, the leader gives verbal input which helps them visualize imaginery objects, refine their actions or get new ideas for deepening or furthering the action. For example, if the leader has asked the players to simultaneously plant a garden in pantomime, he or she might side coach by saying things like, "Feel the hot sun beating down on your neck. Feel the gentle breeze blowing against your cheek. Can you let the soil run through your fingers? What kind of seeds are you planting? What do they feel like?" Verbal answers are not expected for any of the questions. They are asked primarily to stimulate the flow of ideas. The leader's tone of voice needs to be supportive rather than directive and must indicate that no answer is required. This technique is used primarily with pantomime activities when players don't need to get into dialogue.

Modelling. When the leader asks the players to do something, he or she may demonstrate one way it might be done. This is a technique used more often in early sessions to help create a climate of camaraderie and to help allay fears of those who are new to drama and very apprehensive. For example, the leader might say, "Let's get out a bucket of soapy

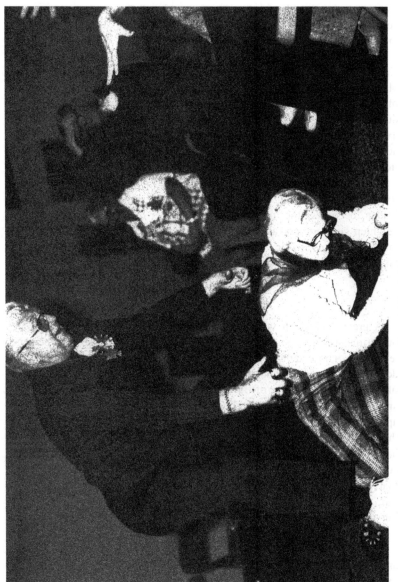

Photo by Dawn Murray

water and clean up the windows in front of us." The leader pantomimes getting a bucket and washing the windows while speaking to guide others to join in the activity.

Spotlighting. At a certain moment the leader may freeze the action in simultaneous play and ask all participants to watch one player, or pair of players, continue action. The leader may then "freeze" that player or players and spotlight someone else. This allows those who are having difficulty getting ideas to gain some inspiration and can be a fun sharing experience. Groups can very briefly share parts of their scenes and characters as they build confidence for longer sharing. **Spotlighting should not be used until players are quite comfortable with each other.**

Leading in Role. This technique allows the leader to stimulate the imaging and believing processes of the participants. For example, the leader "becomes" the tour guide or auctioneer or restaurant *maitre d'* to heighten commitment and stimulate involvement in the drama. Because the leader takes a role, or plays a part, participants are encouraged to take roles as well (see Chapter 7).

Awakening the Senses

A great deal of all we know has come through our senses. They are our primary way of knowing. When the senses are not used they become less acute. Those seniors who live in nursing and convalescent homes are deprived of the warm and pungent smells of their own kitchens, the feel of soil and the fragrance of flowers from their own gardens, and the noise and movement of the neighborhood schoolyard. Even seniors who live in apartments may miss the musty smell of a basement or the dry dust of the attic. It is particularly important for the elderly whose sensory world has shrunk to be exposed to further sensory stimulation. Some of the activities that follow include the presentation of real sensory objects so that participants experience directly the sensations of smell, taste, texture, sounds, etc. Other activities involve sensory recall, i.e., remembering the smell of grandmother's freshly baked bread, the feel of dew-laden grass, the taste of the season's first watermelon.

The decline of sensory function often results in a loss of self-esteem and a feeling of inadequacy. By using sensory recall and direct sensory experience as suggested in the activities that follow, an individual's senses can be awakened to a more responsive level. This can result in an increased confidence in the ability to function in the world.

WHAT A BIG NOSE YOU HAVE, MY DEAR

Objectives: Activate the sense of smell.

Discriminate from among several odors.

Recall images associated with different odors.

Directions: Before the session begins, the leader prepares by putting into bottles and sacks items that have identifiable odors such as limburger cheese, a rose, perfume, cooked cabbage, cinnamon, pepper, orange peel, machine oil, bacon, etc.

Divide group into pairs. One in each pair closes eyes or is blindfolded while the other holds up the bottle or sack containing the odor to be experienced.

The leader reminds the participants that the object of the activity is to experience the odor, recall some association, and not simply to name the odor.

By asking a different question after each odor is presented the leader can challenge participants to go beyond the obvious. Questions can include:

Where might you find this odor? Describe that place to your partner.

Can you remember a specific time you smelled this odor? Tell your partner about it.

Can you remember who you were with when you smelled this odor? Tell your partner.

How many words can you find to describe this odor? Tell them to your partner.

How does this odor make you feel? Tell your partner.

If you were to choose a sound to go with or be like this odor, what might it be?

Materials: Assortment of foods, plants/herbs, toiletries, etc. with identifiable odors placed in bottles or sacks; large plastic prescription bottles work well.

A NEW TWIST ON AN OLD PRETZEL

Objectives: Activate the sense of smell, taste.
Stimulate imagination, practice "what if" thinking.

Directions: Give each person a twisted pretzel and ask him or her to look at it carefully, but not eat it yet. *What might this be other than a pretzel? What does its shape remind you of?* (For example, a bow tie, pair of glasses, peace symbol, butterfly, race track for miniature car, etc.) Get as many responses as possible.

The ask the players to close their eyes and drink in the smell of the pretzel. *What does it remind you of? What do your noses tell you?*

Now, ask the participants to experience the pretzel with the tongue. *Rub the pretzel along your tongue, your lips. What is the first sensation? What is the first taste? The second taste?*

Ask them to take a very little bite and chew slowly. *What do you taste? Keep chewing, but don't swallow. How has the taste changed? How has the texture changed? Is there more saliva? What has happened to the salty taste?* Now ask them to swallow and then enjoy the rest of the pretzel.

Development: The experience may be repeated using an imaginary pretzel to practice the recall of real experience.

The activity may be varied by using other foods, comparing the odor, flavor and texture of apple and cantaloupe for example.

Materials: Box of twisted pretzels.

IT FEELS LIKE

Objectives: Activate the sense of touch.
Extend the sensory vocabulary.

Directions: Before the session begins, the leader assembles a variety of objects that are not easily identified by touch. Objects should vary in size, shape, texture, weight, etc. There should be at least one object for each person in the group.

Divide the group into pairs and ask one player in each pair to close his or her eyes. Place an object in the lap or hands of each non-seeing player and allow all pairs to work simultaneously. The non-seeing player will feel and describe an object to the sighted partner. The goal is *not* to name the object, but to experience and describe it.

Reverse seeing and non-seeing roles and repeat procedure.

Share reactions to the experience discussing which sensations were strange, exciting, tension producing, pleasant, etc.

Materials: Variety of objects: Hats, carvings, macrame, basket, fur parka, candle stick, wallet, Christmas tinsel, rope, doll, strainer, Halloween mask, back brush, stuffed animal, telephone, shoe tree, can opener, artificial flowers, slinky toy, plastic toys, etc.

Development: To challenge the players further and to extend their sensory vocabulary, ask each to contribute a single image for a group poem. For example:

Our Hands Told Us
The slickness of glass
The softness of curtains
The stickiness of a piece of cake
The heat of a lamp.

The images could also be expressed using alliteration. For example:

The gloss of glass
The crispness of curtains

SLEUTH

Objectives: Focus attention on appearance of partner.
Identify changes in appearance of partner.

Directions: Discuss qualities of a good detective with emphasis on the need for keen observation. Talk about other occupations that require keen observation (artist, astronomer, bird watcher, doctor, weatherman).

Have partners sit opposite each other or stand in two lines facing each other. Ask partners to observe each other for 40 seconds, noticing costume, accessories and hairstyle.

At the end of 40 seconds, ask partners to turn their backs on each other and change two or three things about their clothing, hairstyle, etc. (Take off necklace, turn scarf around, put watch on other arm.) When they have had time to complete the change, ask all players to turn again and face their partners. Ask them to observe quietly for a moment, then to share the changes they can detect.

Briefly discuss any funny, unusual or obscure changes.

Materials: The leader may need to provide a box of costume pieces to make this activity more challenging. Suggestions: jewelry, scarves, neckties, hats, etc.

SEE AND REMEMBER

Objectives: Activate powers of observation and recall.
Share and discuss methods of recall.

Directions: Before the group enters, arrange 10 different and interesting objects on a table. Cover objects with a cloth.

Explain to members of the group that they will have
one minute to look at objects under the cloth. They are
to see how many of the objects they can remember.

After one minute of observation, replace the cover on
the table of objects. See how many of the objects the
group, working together, can recall. Discuss the methods they used to remember, such as:

shapes	function/use
color	room/location found
size	age/location

Suggested objects:

lamp	bird cage
apple	hair dryer
plant	bath scales
ball	dog collar
hat	bed pan
pancake turner	tape recorder
soap flakes	calendar
pillow	bunch of radishes

Adaptation: Larger objects will have to be used if the group is
visually impaired or non-ambulatory and less able to
get close to the table.

LEND ME YOUR EARS

Objectives: Differentiate among several sounds.
Associate sounds with ideas and feelings.

Directions: Have the group close their eyes and listen to a sound made by the leader. (Sounds can be made by ringing a bell, beating on a wastebasket, blowing a whistle, tinkling of ice in a glass, playing a record of mysterious sounding music, etc.)

After making each sound, the leader asks different questions. Questions to be asked can include:

Where might you be if you heard this sound?
Who might be making a sound like this?
How does this sound make you feel?
What's going on when you hear this sound?

After each sound and question, allow group members to share their ideas or divide group into pairs. Let the pairs share their responses with each other.

Development: Create a scene based on the most evocative ideas. Create a poem based on the various feeling responses.

Materials: Objects with which to make sounds (bell, pots and spoons, harmonica, glasses filled with water, beans/rice in can, vegetable grater, empty oatmeal box). Recordings of sounds.

Note: If many have hearing impairments, be sure to choose sounds that can be heard.

SOUND TRACK

Objectives: Develop confidence in one's ability to think imaginatively.

Associate sounds with characters, settings and dramatic action.

Directions: Talk about TV shows or films in which music and sound effects have been used to set the mood or heighten the action. (Spy films, chase scenes, quiet scenes like sunrises, fight scenes, etc.)

Leader explains that he or she will produce a sound or some music while the group listens with eyes closed. Participants are to imagine they are watching a film. After they have listened, the leader asks them to share the images that have come to them. For example:

1. *What did you see?*
2. *Where was the scene? Inside? Outside? Ocean? City?*
3. *What was happening? Who was there?*
4. *Was this the beginning, middle or end of the film?*
5. *Does the film have a name?*

At first the images may lack detail, color or intensity. In some cases the images will be static and in other cases quite active. With some sounds the images will be fairly similar, while with other sounds the variety will be quite pronounced. As the leader questions for more details, the images will become richer and more complex.

Development: By asking, *What happened next?*, the leader can help individuals elaborate their images into a whole scene or story.

Materials: Possible sounds for stimulus.

1. Drums, rattles, cymbals, wood blocks and bells.
2. Shake ice cubes in glass or metal container.

3. Strike lower notes on piano with both palms out-spread.
4. Recordings: marches, circus music, sound effects, popular music, symphonies.
5. Human voice making sounds of wind, animals, sirens, etc.

Adaptation: Some groups may respond more readily if the leader provides a frame. The leader may say, *The sound you are about to hear comes from a western (or soap opera, or spy thriller etc.).*

SPLIT FOCUS

Objectives: Exercise concentration, sustain focus of attention and sharpen mental alertness.
Share information about interests, background.
Develop initiative in asking questions.

Directions: Sit or stand in a circle of 7-8 persons. One person, who will be the questioner, stands in the center. The questioner must focus eye contact on the person to whom the question is asked. The addressee must return the gaze but not answer the question. The person to the right of the addressee must answer the question as though it were asked of him or her.

If the addressee answers or laughs, he or she must go into the center of the circle and become the questioner.

If the person to the right does not respond or does so too slowly, he or she must go into the center of the circle and become the questioner.

It is suggested that the leader of the group become the first questioner to get the game off to a vigorous start.

Questions that may be answered *yes* or *no* are disqualified although the leader can ask that they be rephrased, for example:

Did you have a good breakfast this morning?
(yes/no)
What did you eat for breakfast this morning?
(rephrased)

Did you come from a large family?
(yes/no)
How many children were there in your family?
(rephrased)

Other questions that might be asked are:

What did you do Saturday night?

If you could have any job in the world, what would it be?

Where would you like to spend your summer vacation?

Movement and Pantomime

Pain and physical discomfort can affect a person's mental state. Drama cannot reverse the grip of arthritis in the knee, but it can help to make the pain more bearable by encouraging movement in other parts of the body. Many older people have lost their body awareness to such an extent that they have trouble locating their waist, shoulder or elbow. For others, muscles have lost their tone from lack of use. Control and coordination are poor. Bodies are either too relaxed or too tense for good health. These physical conditions are reflected in the facial expression or lack of it, the voice or speech, the thinking processes and attitudes.

Exercises such as yoga and aerobics are helpful to such people and can be found in other books. The activities included here are primarily those that make use of imagery or characterization and deal in some way with the dramatic imagination. Some of the exercises can be done from a sitting position, while others call for participants to stand and move about. But most of the activities can be adapted for those in wheelchairs or with limited movement ability. Almost all of the activities function to raise the energy level, promote coordination and increase body awareness. In addition they serve as a foundation for later work in improvisation.

The leader should know whether a disability is physical or psychological in origin and be guided accordingly. The tendency is to expect too little rather than too much so it's important to remember that most older adults would profit from a greater output of energy.

MIRROR REFLECTION AND STRETCH

Objectives: Develop concentration by focusing on the movements of a partner.
Exercise control of body by working in slow motion.
Stretch and relax muscles of the arms and torso.

Directions: This activity may be done in either a sitting or standing position. Leader asks group to become his or her mirror, following every movement as closely as possible. Leader should use a variety of movement, all in extremely slow motion.

1. Start with a large slow stretch, arch back, hold the stretch for a moment.
2. Follow stretch with a big yawn, throwing the head back, then draw head to chest. Repeat 1 and 2.
3. Stretch the right arm diagonally away from the body. Let arm flop to side.
4. Stretch left arm diagonally away from body. Let arm flop to side.
5. Slowly lean forward and look into mirror, opening eyes widely. Yawn, drooping jaw. Wrinkle nose. Stick out tongue, move it slowly to left and right. Squint eyes tight. Open eyes wide. Move mouth and nose to left, then right.
6. Drop head to chest, then slowly, slowly rotate head to the left, over the shoulder, but do not raise the shoulder to meet the head. Continue head roll, allowing the mouth to open as head tips backward. Continue head roll over other shoulder and allow it to come to rest on the chest. Easy, do not force.

Development: Ask players to take a partner, one partner to be a sleepy person just arising, the other to be the mirror. Players should be in mirror reflection position before starting. Ask the sleepy person to take a starting position and "freeze it." Then ask the mirror to take up that same position and "freeze it." Now in exact mirror relation they are ready to start. Coach players to stay in very slow motion. This should be a silent activity. Talking destroys the concentration.

Suggest that players exchange roles, the mirror becoming the sleepy person and the sleepy person becoming the mirror. When this exercise is working well, it will be difficult to ascertain which is the person and which the mirror.

Other suggested mirror movements include:

     shaving
     putting on make-up
     combing hair
     washing a window
     picking apples
     painting a picture

SHAKE A LEG

Objectives: Exercise all parts of the body.
                  Enjoy relaxing with the group.

Directions: Participants stand far enough apart so they can spread their arms horizontal to the floor without touching anyone else. The leader then gives the following directions, demonstrating as he or she speaks. Everyone participates at the same time.

     1. *Wiggle your fingers. Keep everything else still and just move your fingers. Be relaxed.*
     2. *Now stop wiggling your fingers and just move*

*your hands. Bend at the wrist. Rotate your hands
in a circle. Move gently.*

3. *Now stop your hands and bend at the elbows.
Let your forearms swing back and forth.*
4. *Now move only your shoulders. Up and down.
Around and around. Use relaxed movement.*
5. *Now move your head. Let it sway from side to
side. Gently drop your head to your chest and
slowly rotate it around in a circle.*
6. *Stop your head and get your waist into the action. Bend the upper torso up and down. Rotate
your upper torso.*
7. *Now stop your waist and move at the hips.*
8. *Stop the hips and move at the knees.*
9. *Stop the knees and move at the ankles. Flex
them. Rotate the ankles.*
10. *Now just wiggle your toes.*

After the leader has directed participants to move each
portion of the body separately, he or she can repeat the
activity in a cumulative fashion. In other words, the
leader starts by asking the players to wiggle the fingers,
then to continue wiggling the fingers but also begin to
move the hands. Then to continue both of those motions
but add on movement at the elbow and so forth until
the entire body is in motion.

Adaptation: Non-ambulatory participants can do much of this activity seated in wheelchairs. Only steps 7, 8 and perhaps
9 would have to be eliminated.

ADVERBS

Objectives: Communicate ideas through actions.
              Observe and discriminate among differing qualities of
              movement.

Directions: Divide the group in half. Half "A" decides on an adverb
              keeping it a secret from Half "B." Half "B" thinks up
              several large actions that Half "A" can pantomime.

              The "B" people arrange themselves in a large circle and
              sit down. The "A" people spread out within the circle
              and remain standing.

              One person from "B" calls out a large action for the
              "A" group to perform in the manner of the chosen
              adverb. For example, if the chosen word were *lazily*
              and the action called out was *paint a house*, the "A"
              people would simultaneously pantomime painting a
              house lazily. Note that each player will interpret *paint-
              ing* and *lazily* a bit differently.

              The "B" people observe the pantomimes and try to
              guess the adverb. It is important that no guessing be
              done until the leader gives a signal. Otherwise, guess-
              ing could go on throughout the action destroying con-
              centration. If the first guess is incorrect, another "B"
              person calls out a different action. The "A's" then pan-
              tomime it in the manner of the word, e.g., driving a car
              lazily.

              If the guessing goes on too long and enthusiasm begins
              to lag, the leader can help by telling participants if a
              guess is *close* or *not so close*.

              Once a correct guess has been made, the groups can
              switch. "B" decides on an adverb, and "A" tries to
              guess.

              Large actions might include:

                  Climbing a mountain
                  Digging a hole

Exercising
Washing an elephant

Adverbs that might be used:

sleepily	slowly
angrily	quickly
playfully	sleepily
mysteriously	awkwardly
gloomily	nervously
suspiciously	creatively

Materials: None

PANTOMIME FOR ONE AND TWO

Objectives: Visualize the size, shape and weight of an imagined object.

Communicate a response to an imaginary object.

Work together in a common task without the use of words.

Directions: Leader can introduce the activity by asking the group to watch his or her pantomimed use of an object, such as washing windows with spray bottle and cloth, or putting on make-up using lipstick and mirror. Ask the group to identify the imaginary objects and how they were used to help communicate the action.

The leader should ask the group to really see the objects they use, even though they are not present. As the leader calls out a variety of actions, the group should do their pantomimes simultaneously.

Some sidecoaching during the short pantomimes may be necessary to help the players to establish and sustain their belief. (See p. 24)

Development: Pantomimes that can be done from seated position:

Take a dose of medicine
Try on new tight gloves

Drink a fizzy drink
Shuck corn
Read a newspaper
Play solitaire
Cook flapjacks
Play the piano
Arrange flowers in a bowl
Swat flies
String beads
Thread a needle

Pantomimes that are better done standing:
Shovel snow
Polish a car
Measure for new drapes
Plant flowers
Build a campfire
Walk a dog
Feed the chickens
Fix a leaky faucet
Harness a horse

Spotlighting: After players have become comfortable with each other and no longer feel self-conscious, the leader may use the spotlighting technique (see p. 26). The time allowed for volunteers to show their pantomime should be kept very short.

Variation: After players have developed some confidence and trust in their ability to handle imaginary objects when working alone, ask them to find a partner and a space to move in. Invite all the pairs to work at the same time. Remind them to share the objects and action.

Pantomime for Two:
Hanging wallpaper
Making a bed
Washing the dog
Cleaning the attic
Loading a truck
Moving a piano
Performing an operation

Putting up a tent
Hoisting a sail
Sandbagging a levee
Tasting tea or wine
Birdwatching with one pair of binoculars
Playing checkers or chess
Washing and drying dishes

STATUE MAKER

Objectives: Explore posture, gesture and facial expression as a means of communication.
Use the sense of touch to give and receive information.
Create three-dimensional images with the body.

Directions: Talk about any statues that are familiar to the group (Statue of Liberty, Venus di Milo, Flag Raising at Iwo Jima, Michaelangelo's David, etc.). Discuss why the sculptor often uses a live model to help determine the desired pose.

Ask each person to find a partner. One is to be the sculptor, the other will be the model. The model must let the sculptor move her or him about until the right pose is found. All sculptors will work simultaneously.

The leader will give a title for the statue as a starting point. Some titles might be:
Scarlett O'Hara at the Ball
The Dragon Cornered
Skydiver
The Mad Scientist
Man Overboard
The Arsonists
Betsy Ross Makes a Flag
David Before Goliath
Scarecrow at Work
The Thinker
Finding Baby Moses in the Bullrushes

When the statues are finished, ask each sculptor to make some brief comments about the new masterpiece.

Development: Polaroid photographs can record the poses of the statues and the feeling of the sculptor towards his statue. The photographs could be displayed along with the title of the statue.

Note: This activity can be tiring for the model if allowed to go on for too long. Urge the sculptors to work quickly. May be difficult if both partners are in wheelchairs.

1-2-3-SHAPE

Objectives: Overcome self-consciousness about body image.
Limber the body through changing body positions and shapes.
Use kinesthetic response to shape as an impetus to the creation of a character.

Directions: Leader asks group members to distribute themselves throughout the playing area. They are to move through space, to push through space using arms and the whole body as the leader says *1-2-3* very slowly. Upon hearing, *Shape*, the players stop and hold their position.

The *1-2-3 Shape* is repeated several times. At one time the group is asked to use their bodies to make curved lines and shapes, at another, straight lines and angles. They are encouraged to work at different levels, high, medium and low. Leader reminds them of various body parts to use: head, elbows, knees, hips, etc. They can be encouraged to try shapes that are funny, ugly, scary, tense, droopy.

Development: After working with curving lines and shapes and holding a frozen position, the leader asks players to imagine they are a flower, tree or other plant. They are asked to stay in one place, but to move as that plant. Questions that can stimulate thoughtful participation are: *Is your flower strong? weak? hot? thirsty? How does it respond to the sun? the wind? the rain? What kind of flower are you?* Players are to respond in movement to the questions, not answer verbally.

After working with angular lines and shapes and holding a frozen position, the leader asks players to imagine they are some kind of animal. They are asked to move as that animal. Suggestions for side coaching: *What is your animal about to do? Is it looking for something? Is it afraid of something? What might it find? What kind of animal are you?*

After working with both angular and curved movement and taking a frozen position, the leader asks players to imagine that they are a statue about to come to life. *What kind of statue are you? What is your statue about to do next? Where is it—in a park? in a museum? What problem does your statue have? Bring your statue back to rest in a frozen pose.*

Spotlighting: Leader may ask if some players would share their movement ideas. *Would a few share the flower movement? Animal? Statue?*

Adaptation: This activity can be adapted for people in wheelchairs by concentrating on movement of the arms, head, neck and upper torso.

FREEZE IT!

Objectives: Discover and express ideas spontaneously while moving, not before moving.

Trust and respond to first impulses.

Develop flexible thinking in responding to a variety of stimuli.

Develop greater freedom in expressing ideas with the whole body.

Directions: Leader introduces the activity while players are seated. Players are asked to respond with the first word/words that come to mind when the leader says a single word, i.e., "Rainbow" or "Alarm Clock." Go around the room quickly, trying to get a response from each person, but allowing a player to say "pass" if he or she cannot think of a response at the time. Come back to those persons later. Comment on the variety of ideas expressed and the strength and color of the images. Choose a few of the responses and discuss how they might be translated into action.

Briefly discuss the kind of movement players might use upon hearing the following words:

Leaves: raking leaves, pressing leaves in a book, cleaning leaves in gutter

Kitchen: baking a cake, washing dishes, frying pancakes

Mosquito: trying to find one in the dark, putting lotion on bites

Leader indicates that it's important to trust that first idea, that first impression and translate it into movement for the next part of the activity.

Ask participants to take a space in the room where they will not bump into anyone. As leader calls out one word at a time, players respond simultaneously in pantomime, paying no attention to anyone else in the room and following their own impulses and ideas. 10-15 seconds after calling out the words, the leader calls

FREEZE IT at which time all players should stop and hold the pose for a couple of seconds. Leader then calls *THAW* and proceeds to the next word.

During the 10-15 seconds of movement, leader may need to remind players to trust their own ideas, to use all the space, to focus their attention on their own action, to refrain from talking and to pay attention to no one else. During the "thaw" period, the group may need to be reminded that there is no right or wrong way to interpret words, each person's way is valid. The leader may also wish to point out the many, many interpretations that were given.

Choose 5-6 words from the different categories listed below for each playing of FREEZE IT.

PLACE WORDS	PEOPLE WORDS
Kitchen*	Dentist*
Library*	Fisherman*
Zoo	Fortune Teller*
Movie theatre*	Shoe clerk
Circus	Juggler*
Park	Baby sitter*
Pet shop*	Gold prospector

SITUATIONS	OBJECTS
Picket Line	Flashlight*
Rummage Sale*	Alarm Clock*
Robbery*	Camera*
Auto accident	Garden tools*
Forest Fire	Hope Diamond*
Stuck elevator*	Telephone*
Hurricane	Make-up Kit*

Adaptation: Players in wheelchairs will be able to respond to most of the words above. An asterisk(*) indicates those activities most easily done by players in wheelchairs.

Development: After the group is able to concentrate on their own actions while pantomiming simultaneously with others, the leader may introduce the following transition into improvisation.

After the group has completed their FREEZE IT pantomime to one of the following cue words, the leader can ask each player to find a partner. They are to work together using dialogue to explore the given situation. All pairs in the group are to work out their scenes at the same time. They may or may not show their scenes to the rest of the group later.

SITUATIONS FOR TWO

Cue Word:	*Situation:*
Secretary	One has just been fired, the other has just received a raise.
Flashlight	Two spies are inside the Pentagon when suddenly the flashlight goes out.
Fortune Teller	Fortune teller has some bad news and some good news for the client.
Pet Shop	A pet shop owner is teaching a new helper how to care for the animals when a boa constrictor arrives.
Dentist's Office	A telephone operator has come to complain about her new upper plate. This is the first set made by the dentist.
Rummage Sale	Two people claim to have seen a certain object first. Each tries to prove his needs are greater.

Stretching the Imagination

Seniors are constantly faced with the need to stretch the dollar but are less likely to see the need to stretch the imagination. For many, work was at the center of their lives before retirement or infirmity. There was little talk of leisure and less of play. Imagination was used in practical ways to solve problems but was rarely used for pure pleasure. Yet, like a muscle, the imagination atrophies if it is not exercised.

Through dramatic activities, seniors can experience an imaginative high, an exhilaration in the moment, an enchantment of being. Wearing the spectacles of imagination, looking with the mind's eye, leads to an exciting kind of inner growth. Impulses, long denied or locked up, are released and trusted. Ideas, previously thought too ridiculous, burst forth producing delight and amazement. Associations never thought of before collide, creating fresh images of beauty and humor. Memories long forgotten make their appearance with vividness and joy.

Drama can precipitate this kind of explosion when participants are asked to recall moments of strong feeling, like their first date. Or they may be invited to associate unrelated objects or people (what could Gloria Swanson and Miss America 1980 talk about?). Participants may be encouraged to identify with another person through "as if" thinking (feed a baby "as if" you were a new mother). Or they may engage in fantasy (how did you discover a way to teach butterflies to read?).

In stretching the imagination, the leader does not ask questions with right or wrong answers but those which elicit the greatest number of possible answers. The leader encourages the flow of ideas, originality, humor, playfulness and flexibility to build the courage and creativity of the group. The leader and participants deal not only with what is, but what might be within the realm of possibility.

TRANSFORMATION OF REAL OBJECTS

Objectives: Use the imagination in the transformation of objects.
Communicate through pantomime.
Observe and identify the object used by others in the group.

Directions: Leader chooses a real object, e.g., paper plate, to be used in the transformation activity. Its normal, accepted use is identified, i.e., a paper plate is for holding food. But the leader suggests that it could have other uses and asks players to watch and guess while he or she uses plate as a frisbee or sunshade.

The leader now passes the object around the circle so participants can show their ideas for transforming the plate. This method serves as a mild press for total participation. So that the press is not too great, individuals may say, *pass*, if they cannot think of an idea at the moment. After the circle has been completed, leader should give those who passed another chance.

If a player's pantomime is unclear, the leader may ask that it be repeated or may use questions to help the player clarify his or her actions.

Materials: Suggested objects for the activity:

Yardstick	Step ladder
Length of rope	Wastebasket
Crepe paper streamer	Length of colored fabrics
L'egg eggs	

Participants might transform a yardstick as follows:

Baton	Flute
Telescope	Baseball bat
Fishing pole	Violin bow
Rifle	Boat paddle
Umbrella	Sword
Spade	Rolling pin
Cane	Rug beater

PRECIOUS OBJECTS: WHAT PEOPLE VALUE

Objectives: Associate attributes of an object with a particular character.

Communicate a relationship toward a particular object.

Use imagination to explore various dimensions of character (age, occupation, attitude, goals, hobbies, values).

Directions: Before beginning the session, the leader arranges a variety of objects (a few more than the number of participants) on the table. Ask group members to observe the objects closely and choose one that interests or intrigues him or her.

The leader asks each participant to decide on a character who might have made the object, or who owns the object. In any case, the object must have some special significance or value for the character.

To help participants add dimension to their characters, the leader can ask them to consider the following:

1. *Is your character living today or did he or she live years ago?*
2. *In what country is your character living?*
3. *What is your character's occupation?*
4. *Is your character rich or poor?*
5. *Does your character drive a Mercedes, ride a bicycle or what?*
6. *Is your character an orphan or from a large family?*
7. *Where did you get this object? How long have you had it?*
8. *Why is it so important to you? Would you sell it?*
9. *Has anything unusual happened to you and this object?*
10. *What difficulties or problems has this object caused you?*
11. *If this object could talk, what would the two of you talk about?*

These questions need not be answered aloud. The leader may just request that each person answer them for him or herself.

After giving the group thinking time, the leader announces that all have been chosen to be interviewed on a new TV show called PRECIOUS OBJECTS: WHAT PEOPLE VALUE.

Divide into groups of 4-5, assigning a master of ceremonies for each group. The master of ceremonies will interview each character asking such questions as:

How did you come into possession of this object?
How long have you owned the object?
Why is it important to you?
Can you tell us any problems you have had concerning this object?

Note that open questions will draw out more information, but some people may have to be helped with more specific questions.

With some groups it might be better not to sub-divide, working all together with the leader as the master of ceremonies.

FORTUNATELY/UNFORTUNATELY

Objectives: Practice flexible thinking and image formation.
Enjoy one's own cleverness and the cleverness of others.

Directions: The group sits in a circle. The leader starts a story beginning with the word *fortunately*. The person sitting next to the leader must continue the story, but his or her first word must be *unfortunately*. The story is built sentence by sentence. The sentences alternately begin with the words *fortunately* and *unfortunately*, as each person in the circle takes a turn.

For example:

Leader: *Fortunately, I won a vacation to the Everglades.*
Person 2:   *Unfortunately, I fell into the swamp.*
Person 3:   *Fortunately, I could swim.*
Person 4:   *Unfortunately, a crocodile saw me swimming.*
Person 5:   *Fortunately, I saw a stick in the water and grabbed it and jammed it between the jaws of the crocodile.*
Person 6:   *Unfortunately, it wasn't a stick at all, but a snake meditating.*

The story continues as each person takes a turn. Note that the responses are only one sentence in length. This is important so the story keeps building and also because the suddenness of the story twists adds to the enjoyment.

WOULD YOU BELIEVE?

Objectives: Relax and trust oneself in a playful situation.
Develop fluency of ideas and spontaneity of expression.
Develop "as if" thinking through a fantasy experience
in which the illogical is treated as logical.

Directions: Ask group to find partners. In pairs they are to take
turns in telling each other all about one of the following
(include as many details as can be remembered):

1. Something they did over the weekend.
2. An interesting show they saw on TV.
3. A funny thing that has happened to them.
4. An event that surprised or shocked them, etc.

Development: Next they are to come up with the biggest "whopper"
they can imagine, but they must convince their partner
that it really happened. A few examples may help to
stretch their imaginations.

1. *The day I stood in for Greta Garbo or Mae West.*
2. *How I make clothes out of seaweed.*
3. *I live in a house the size of a sugar cube.*
4. *My grandmother owned the Hope diamond.*
5. *I fly south with the robins each fall.*
6. *My doctor has X-Ray fingers.*
7. *I cooked dinner for the King of the Hobos.*
8. *I grow spaghetti on the roof of my house.*
9. *I trained Joe Louis.*
10. *My twin sons climbed Mt. Everest.*
11. *How to cheat at Bingo.*

Ground rule: The listening partner may ask a few questions, but should not dominate the narration. Above all,
he or she may not disbelieve the "whopper." The listener's belief and interest will strongly support the teller's
efforts to act "as if" it really happened.

Discussion: 1. *What did your partner do or say that made you believe his or her "big whopper?"*

2. *What was the funniest or most outlandish thing your partner said?*
3. *What helped you to believe in your own whopper?*
4. *Can you think of any famous authors who made a whopper into a story?* (Mark Twain, "Jumping Frog of Calavaras County," O. Henry, "Cop and the Anthem")

HOW'S THAT?

Objectives: Become aware of simple story structure, i.e., beginning, middle and end.
Use imagination to justify and link seemingly unrelated ideas.
Practice flexible thinking and image formation.

Directions: The group sits in a circle. The leader begins a story. The next person says a word that is seemingly unrelated to the story. The third person must continue the story begun by the leader, but incorporate the second person's word within the story. The fourth person says another word. The fifth person continues the story including the fourth person's word. This pattern continues around the circle, with the leader ending the story.

For example:

Leader: *Once upon a time a little green dwarf lived deep in the forest. One day he felt very adventurous, and so, for the first time, he walked to the town on the edge of the forest. He wandered among the people. Almost immediately the town folk began to gather around the dwarf . . . "Poor little boy," someone said. "Why are you all alone? Are you an orphan? Where are your mother and father?" The dwarf was puzzled. "What's a mother and father?" he asked. When the town folk told him, the little green dwarf decided it would be very nice to have parents. So he set out on a journey into the world seeking the whereabouts of his own mother and father.*

(Note that the leader provided (1) a leading character who (2) has a problem and goal and (3) a particular place to start from.)

Person 2:   (States a word seemingly unrelated to the story.) *Popcorn.*

Person 3:   (Must relate the word "popcorn" to the story in two to four sentences.) *As the little green dwarf walked down the road, he realized how hungry he was. "How good some popcorn would taste right now," he thought, but all he had was a crust of bread in his pocket.*

Some words that might be used are:

stomachache	dictionary
midnight	suspenders
pitchfork	earthquake
magician	sardines
Grand Canyon	home

The first time this activity is tried, the leader may wish to give out a card (to every other person) on which a word has previously been written. This can assure a greater variety of stimulus and promote more imagination leaps in relating unrelative ideas.

Development: Other stories the leader might begin are:

1. *It was a bad day in the flying carpet factory. None of the carpets would fly. The owner called all the workers together and told them no one was leaving until they discovered why the carpets would not fly.*

2. *Detective Cribbage was frantic. He was called in to investigate the murder of Ms. Pip in Room 41X of*

the Merry Hours Motel, a sleazy dump on the south side of town. In Ms. Pip's pockets was a note from the murderer saying Detective Cribbage was next. Detective Cribbage was frantic. He had to find the murderer—and fast!

Materials: Cards with words (see above)

TWENTY QUESTIONS: WHO AM I?

Objectives: Recall details of events and lives of famous people. Participate in group discussion and decision making. Concentrate and listen actively.

Directions: One person in the group is selected to go out of the room and be "it." The others then decide on a famous person that "it" is supposed to be. "It" returns and begins asking "yes" or "no" questions to discover who he or she is. "It" is allowed twenty questions.

The leader must make certain that "it" phrases the questions so they can be answered with a *yes* or *no*. (*Am I living or dead?* is an illegal question because it cannot be answered with a *yes* or *no*. *Am I dead?* is allowable.)

Another person is selected to be "it" when the first person either guesses his or her identity correctly or has asked a total of twenty questions.

It is important that the group agree they have enough information about the famous person before a final selection is made so that "its" questions can be answered correctly.

To simplify the game for the early rounds, the leader may identify the category for "it" by announcing at the outset, *You are a famous sports figure*. Another way of simplifying the game is to simply limit selection to one category. For example, one day all the famous

people must be outlaws, while another day they may all
be explorers.

Development: Possible categories and persons:

Inventors:	Thomas Alva Edison, Henry Ford, Alexander Graham Bell
Political:	Bella Abzug, Eleanor Roosevelt, Fiorello LaGuardia
Outlaws:	Al Capone, Jesse James, Ma Barker
Sports:	Babe Ruth, Knute Rockne, Babe Diedrickson Zaharias
Explorers:	Columbus, Marco Polo, Admiral Byrd
Entertainers:	Pavlova, Jenny Lind, P. T. Barnum
Biblical:	Noah, Moses, Judas
Fictional:	Scrooge, Peter Pan, Scarlet O'Hara

ODD-U-PATIONS

Objectives: Develop image making ability and descriptive vocabulary.

Enjoy playful situations, ridiculous ideas.

Find logic in the illogical.

Develop creative thinking by making the strange seem normal.

Directions: Two people select one of the weird occupations below or create one of their own.

Leader introduces the pair to the group as the only people in the world with their occupation. They are very successful, business is booming and they are desperate to entice more people into this occupation. They have come to make explanations and to answer questions. The leader may kick things off by taking a role first, answering questions and then solicit questions from the group.

The trick and challenge is to treat a ridiculous possibility as an accomplished fact. A serious attitude and straight face as well as nimble thought are required to fully enjoy this activity.

POSSIBLE ODD-U-PATIONS

Teaching butterflies to read
Developing a way of getting hens to lay hardboiled eggs
Making jet brooms for witches in a hurry
Training boa constrictors to squeeze orange juice
Inventing a way to straighten the tails of pigs
Unionizing termites as building wreckers
Discovering a method to help squirrels locate buried nuts
Providing legal aid for cockroaches

EYEWITNESS

Objectives: Tell a story from the perspective of a specific role.

Exercise "as if" thinking; project self into imagined event.

Develop a role and help other players by asking appropriate questions.

Recall pertinent and relevant information from past experience.

Directions: 3-4 people select an event from the list below or agree on one of their own choosing. They are to imagine they have just come from witnessing that event and are now appearing before a group of newspersons who are preparing stories for their papers.

The leader takes the role of head of the Associated Press Bureau who moderates the press conference, allowing the eyewitnesses to describe all they can remember and encouraging the rest of the group as news reporters to ask questions so the full story may be revealed. Witnesses are free to show or demonstrate some part of their narrative.

To help the news reporters believe in their role, the leader can give each a card to identify his or her newspaper: New York Times, Washington Post, Chicago Tribune, Los Angeles Examiner, etc.

Allow time for eyewitnesses and reporters to meet. Eyewitnesses should pool their information about the event. Reporters should formulate some questions for the interview.

Leader must treat the inquiry with absolute sincerity, using his or her role to increase the belief. Leader must be ready with questions to ask the witnesses and be prepared to help the newspersons in the phrasing of their questions.

POSSIBLE EVENTS

(Some events occurred within the lifetime of the players, some did not.)

> Charles Lindberg Arrives in New York
> Sinking of the Titanic
> Abdication of Edward VIII
> Alaskan Gold Rush
> San Francisco Earthquake
> Custer's Last Stand
> Burning of Atlanta
> Building of Noah's Ark
> Jesse Owens at Berlin Olympics
> VE or VJ Days
> Civil Rights Marches
> Building of Hoover Dam
> Women Get the Vote
> Chicago Fire
> Discovery of King Tut's Tomb
> Neil Armstrong Lands on Moon
> Driving the Golden Spike
> Columbus Discovers America
> Gertrude Ederle Swims English Channel

Materials: Cards with the name of a different newspaper on each.

DOWN MEMORY LANE #1

Objectives: Reawaken memories of past experiences, particularly those of childhood and youth.

Listen with great concentration to a partner.

Share personal thoughts in close intimate relationship.

Directions: While group is gathering, play a recording of the song "Memories" or pass out copies of the words and sing the song together.

Before starting the activity, talk about memories. Some questions might include:

1. *Why are some memories stronger than others?*
2. *What faces can you see most clearly?*
3. *What places are most vivid in your mind?*
4. *Which events from your childhood seem like they happened yesterday?*

Some memories are tiny fragments, a face, a voice. Some are compact and distilled like poetry. Some memories are more complete like a story with a beginning, middle and end.

To get the activity started, arrange group in pairs. Partners should be sitting quite close to each other with some space between the pairs. Ask each pair to decide which is A and which is B. A will start as the "rememberer" while B is the "listener." The rememberer may feel more comfortable with his or her eyes closed. Unless the rememberer needs some encouragement, the listener should do just that—listen.

The leader will give a memory starter (see below) which is to be repeated by B to A. All B's will repeat the starter simultaneously and all B's will listen while all A's do their remembering simultaneously. After 3-4 minutes, the leader will give another starter.

MEMORY STARTERS by leader and repeated by B to A:

1. *Tell me about all the tastes you can remember from childhood.*
2. *Tell me about your favorite family vacation.*
3. *Tell me about someone you were afraid of as a child.*
4. *Tell me about your favorite friend in high school.*
5. *Tell me about a family wedding you attended.*

After A has reminisced about the above subjects, A becomes the listener and B the rememberer. The leader gives a different set of starters this time.

MEMORY STARTERS said by leader and repeated by A to B:

1. *Tell me about all the smells you can remember from childhood.*
2. *Tell me about your first date.*
3. *Tell me about your grandmother/grandfather.*
4. *Tell me about your favorite teacher.*
5. *Tell me about a holiday or special family celebration.*

The starters should relate to the kind of experience almost everyone has had and no attempt should be made to plumb deeply the depths of traumatic experiences like accidents, serious illness, death or divorce.

Chapter 4

LEADING THE WAY

Leader Behavior

Perhaps the key ingredient in the success of creative drama sessions, besides careful planning, is the behavior of the leader. If you are friendly, organized and warm, the sessions are much more likely to be successful than if you are disorganized and distant. If you have a positive attitude about the drama sessions, the participants are much more likely to enjoy and look forward to the sessions. If you are sincere in the interest you show each participant and in the enthusiasm you show for each activity, you will have far more success than a leader who is dispirited, disinterested or bored. There are specific things one can do to improve leadership. Following is a discussion of some of them.

1. *Be warm, friendly, and above all, enthusiastic.* If you have a good time, the participants are likely to have a good time. If you make them feel welcome, they will want to come back. On days when you are down, make the effort to behave in an enthusiastic manner and you are likely to find that you soon truly feel the same way. Enthusiasm, even deliberate enthusiasm, is contagious.

2. *Know and use each person's name.* Take the time to personally greet each resident as they enter and before they leave. Compliment them on their contributions. Be specific. Look forward to seeing them next time. Remember what they did in the last session. Develop their trust in you. Take the time to show you notice and care.

3. *Establish physical contact.* A touch on the shoulder, a gentle squeeze on the arm, holding someone's hand all say, "I care, I think you're important, I want to be your friend." Physical contact helps to develop a supportive trusting atmosphere, especially for those with poor eyesight and/or hearing.

4. *Maintain strong eye contact.* Looking people in the eye when you

talk to them makes them feel that you mean what you say, that you really care, that you are totally engaged. Looking someone in the eye when they speak to you demonstrates that you are really listening. Eye contact is crucial to maintaining attention, and it is much more difficult for participants to refuse participation if you look right at them. Remember, though, to share eye contact with the group so no one feels excluded.

5. *Approach participants as your intellectual equals.* Adults, senior adults especially, do not like to be treated like children. You are **not** their teacher, you are simply the leader in a group of peers. Lead with humor and motivation, not authoritarianism. **Nothing can be deadlier than condescension**.

6. *Choose materials with care.* Materials should stimulate the mind, encourage decision making and allow for problem-solving. Many seniors have few decisions left to them. Drama can allow them to regain some measure of control. Choose materials you can personally get excited about. Don't choose something just because someone else said it was a good idea. If you are excited about the materials, participants are likely to be too. If you are lukewarm about it, so will they be. Work with the element of surprise. If you continue to repeat something just because it worked once, not only will you be bored, but so will participants. It is important to choose new materials, new approaches for each lesson.

7. *Overplan.* Be prepared with more material than you think can be covered in one session. It's like an insurance policy. Nothing is worse than running out of material when there is still fifteen minutes of a session left, especially when you're a newcomer to creative drama. If one activity isn't working well, you have another ready in your pocket.

8. *Use a variety of stimuli.* Appeal to the senses, to the imagination and to reason. Props can be useful to you. Use large photographs, colorful prints from the library, concrete objects, bottled scents, food—anything that will assist you in getting and holding attention and drawing forth many responses. Don't forget that questions are also a source of stimulation.

9. *Give clear directions.* This will help take the fear out of the situation for participants. If they know what you are asking them to do, it will be easier for them to participate. If they are unsure what it is you are asking for, they are much more likely to hold back. This means your directions must be crystal clear in your own mind.

10. *Introduce some problem, some conflict into each lesson.* Not only is conflict, tension, suspense, the stuff that drama is made of, but also it serves as a strong motivational device. If nothing is at stake, who cares?

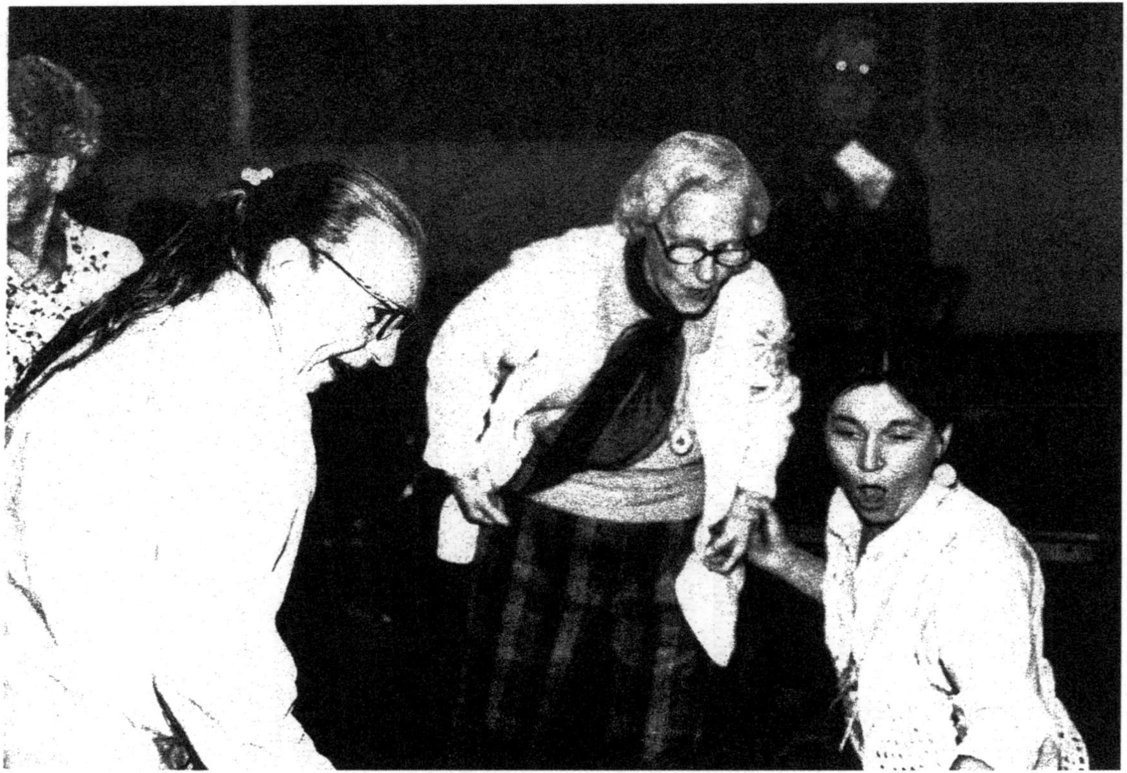

Photo by Dawn Murray

But if there is some question about the outcome, that becomes a different matter. Conflict encourages emotional involvement, stimulates difference of opinion, allows for looking at values and meaning, and deepens the experience for participants.

11. *Use your voice, your face, your whole body as expressive instruments.* Movement not only attracts attention, it also conveys a great deal of meaning. If you move or speak in a lethargic manner, you are conveying lack of interest. If you move with a spring and bounce, you indicate joy and commitment. Your voice and facial expression can communicate warmth, joy and fun, heighten excitement, or connote fear or despair. But remember that a well timed pause, a moment of stillness, attracts attention and provides a focus.

12. *Be ready to share your own experiences.* Telling about your joys, problems or frustrations can serve as a model. If participants hear you opening up, they are more likely to share their experiences. If they see you as a human being, they are more likely to feel comfortable around you. At the same time your sharing should not be heavy handed or take the place of centering the drama on the participant's ideas and experiences. It is meant to stimulate, not stifle or dominate.

13. *Deal in specifics, not generalities.* Use imagination to visualize and communicate a picture, feeling, mood or character. Describe the house, picnic grounds or restaurant in vivid detail so all can see it in their mind's eye. Through questions, lead the group to visualize the details of the blacksmith shop, lighthouse or the bull fight.

14. *Change stimuli and pace frequently.* Watch for signs of boredom. Do not use simple warm-ups or ice breakers for more than five or ten minutes. Do not engage in vigorous exercise for more than a few minutes at a time.

15. *Cultivate openness and flexibility.* Be ready for and value unexpected responses. They are often the mark of creativity. Enjoy surprises. Turn an unrelated or irrelevant response to advantage. Accept all responses sincerely and with good humor. In the eyes of participants, rejecting the response can be seen as a rejection of the person.

16. *Praise, encourage, reinforce all efforts of the group.* Strongly communicate your belief to them and in them. In educational circles there is a phenomenon known as the Pygmalion effect which states that people will behave in a manner concomitant with your expectations of them. If you think they will fail, they will. If you expect them to participate, they will. Create a climate in which risk taking is valued and where there are no right or wrong responses, e.g., ask open-ended questions.

17. *Keep the interest of the whole group.* Don't give in to the temptation to go off on a tangent with Mrs. Jones while everyone else must wait. Avoid allowing one person to dominate. Repeat or relate the contribution of each person back to the drama and to the whole group. Try to get as many responses as possible and don't always call on the same person. From time to time you may have to interrupt a long winded response, summarize a bit and rejoin the direction of the discussion.

18. *Be prepared for interruptions, members arriving late, sudden changes in physical or emotional reactions.* You can preplan what you want to say and do. You can even pre-plan what you hope will be the reactions of your group. But you cannot and should not force reactions or participation. You will have much better cooperation if you respect each individual in the group as a unique adult rather than expecting him or her to behave in some preconceived manner. Doing this requires flexibility, adjustment and creativity on the part of the leader and can lead to great growth for the leader as well.

19. *Use people from outside the group as assistants to play a role whenever it is helpful.* Sometimes another leader or guest may be asked to take a part in the drama as an angry citizen, immovable magistrate or lost stranger to add tension and serve as a point of focus for the drama.

Handling Common Problems

There are always unexpected problems when groups of individuals meet for creative drama but many problems may be resolved by careful advance planning. And while there is always a danger in labeling, we all know that certain types of participant behavior, such as negativism, bossiness or shyness, can make it more difficult for the leader to provide a successful drama experience for everyone in the group. A danger in labels, of course, is that having labeled a person as a certain behavior or personality type, we may cease seeing that individual as a person. Certainly Mrs. Jones might be very bossy, but she undoubtedly has other personality traits as well. Labeling her as bossy, we may fail to see that she is also very bright, has a good sense of humor, is afraid of insects and has a great deal of energy. Having labeled her as bossy, we may view her every act in that context. It is essential that we remind ourselves that a person, while perhaps manifesting some behavior difficult to deal with, has a whole spectrum of personality traits, responses, emotions and needs. We can often work on a negative or disruptive trait through other positive traits. The label is only a handle. We must look at the behavior and its effect on the group without discounting the person.

With that warning in mind, then, let us consider some kinds of behavior that can cause problems, realizing that the behavior is not the person.

The Reluctant Participant

A good number of those who participate in drama groups for senior citizens grew up in a time when traditional roles were much more firmly established than they are today. Men weren't supposed to cry. Women were supposed to be homemakers. Children played. Adults didn't. Pretending was for kids and to be forgotten after that. The ways in which an adult was to behave were more firmly prescribed than is currently true. Adults, particularly senior adults, were to be reserved and dignified and it is difficult for many brought up in such a way to leap into being characters from a circus, for example, without some reluctance. Providing seniors with the opportunity to experience drama is not enough. We must also make it acceptable to enjoy that experience.

We may need to sell our groups on the power of imagination and creativity. For participants brought up on the work ethic and practical things, creative drama may at first seem superfluous. If we can draw a parallel, however, between the creative problem solving and imaginative skills used in the home, the laboratory or the business world with the creative drama process, participants may begin to see that there is some use, some reason for drama as an activity. Once they see some practical value in participating, it may gradually become all right to have a good time participating as well. It is almost as though we must provide a license to fantasize, a license to play, a license to let loose. We must sometimes go slow if we want to reach our goal because we may be working against years of prejudice towards play.

There are other common fears that get in the way of joyous participation: fear of being laughed at, fear of being thought too forward, fear of losing one's dignity, fear of failure, fear of trying new things, fear of the unknown, fear of change, fear of making mistakes. We all experience those fears from time to time, especially in a new and unfamiliar situation, and it is important for the leader to respect the reality of those fears on the part of participants and not to discount their validity. At the same time there are things that the leader can do to help participants to overcome their fears.

One of the most important things a leader can do is to model the

Photo by Dawn Murray

desired behavior. If we want to encourage people to participate in a joyous, free manner, then we must demonstrate positive, outgoing, almost adventurous behavior. If we are diffident, quiet and withdrawn, hesitant to ask for too much or to suggest certain kinds of activities because they seem "silly," how can we expect participants to demonstrate behavior that is any different?

The atmosphere of the group is important as well. There must be no censure, ridicule, competition or comparison. Saying, "No! No! That's all wrong!" to Mrs. Harrison who had to muster every bit of courage she had simply to attempt an exercise could send her back to her protective shell of non-participation for good. There must be a feeling of mutual trust, acceptance and support, and both eye contact and touch can be important here. Looking into Mr. Jones' eyes with a friendly smile and taking him by the hand while saying, "Oh, Mr. Jones, will you be my partner?" can give him the assurance that he needs to feel he can try.

Lack of pressure is important also. Those who are self-conscious need more time before they feel comfortable actively participating. They may need to watch and enjoy passively for a bit before they take the plunge. Or, particularly in a game situation, they may not think they have an idea good enough to offer. In the latter case, it is important for them to have the option of passing.

Nothing can be more deadly than thinking you have to get up in front of the whole group to do a pantomime or speak extemporaneously while everyone's eyes are on you. "Mrs. Johnson, will you please come up here and pantomime planting and watering a garden," is more likely to send Mrs. Johnson quickly to her room than to stimulate her to participate in a drama group, especially in the first few sessions.

On the other hand, inviting everyone in the whole group to participate simultaneously takes the pressure off because it takes the focus off of the individual. "Imagine that we are all gardeners. You are preparing the soil to plant your bean seeds. Be sure you cover them up with enough dirt." Now Mrs. Johnson doesn't have to do her pantomime in front of anyone, because everyone is doing it. Everyone can participate without being on the spot.

Another way the leader can draw out reluctant participants is to directly question them in the most nonthreatening way possible. Mr. Edwards may be dying to put in his two cents, but finds it difficult to take the initiative. A simple question directly put may help him take the plunge. "Do you like to start the day with coffee or tea, Mr. Edwards?" or "Where did you go on your honeymoon?" The sensitivity of the leader is important here.

Other times positive reinforcement or acknowledgement of the least effort can be the key. Praise overdone can be embarrassing and can, in fact, inhibit involvement. But sincere praise for an interesting idea, an honest effort, or participation where there was none before can make someone of any age more anxious to "keep up the good work." We all like to feel we are noticed, that we are appreciated, and that we are capable. We are all more likely to cooperate with the person who stimulates those feelings in us than with a person who sends us vibrations of indifference, or worse, criticism. Open ended questions having no right or wrong answers can be helpful here.

An often overlooked technique for making people feel comfortable, for drawing them out, is for leaders to lower their status a bit. Leaders who can tell stories on themselves, who can make mistakes, who do not know everything, are much more human and effective leaders than those who are super-efficient and seemingly perfect. This is not to say that you should give the impression of being disorganized, scatterbrained or incompetent, but rather that you are comfortable enough to occasionally say, "Boy, I really goofed that one up," or "Could somebody help me get this tape recorder going? I don't seem to be doing it right." The implication to participants, especially those who are afraid or reluctant, is, "If the leader can make a mistake and admit it, I guess I don't have to worry about everything I do being just right."

Hand in hand with this is the ability to laugh at yourself and to have fun with the drama sessions. If leaders are able to laugh with (not at) participants, they help to create a climate of enjoyment.

To encourage participation, it is important that the leader give clear directions. Mrs. Wozniak is much less likely to join in if she is not certain what is expected of her. A direction like, "Move to the music," is fairly vague and not likely to generate much response. Compare it to a direction like the following: "In a moment I am going to play a piece of music. Let's all just close our eyes and listen to it. I'd like you to imagine what kind of creature might enjoy moving about to this music.

"Good. Now that you've heard the music, let's hear your ideas. What kind of creature did you imagine? A butterfly? A hummingbird? Let's try moving our arms like the wings of a butterfly. Good, Charley! Excellent, Helen. Now let's imagine we've come to rest on a warm stone in the sunshine. Now let's try it with the music."

In the second example, the leader is being specific. Clear goals have

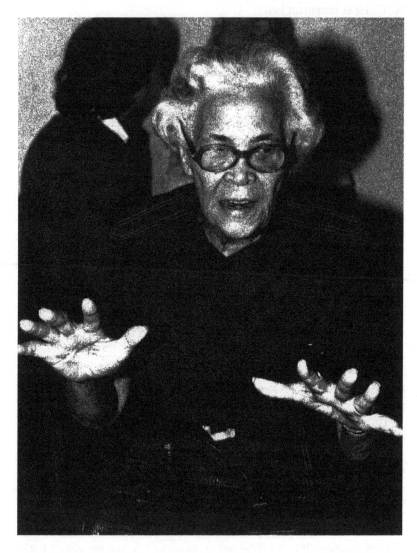

Photo by Dawn Murray

been stated for participants. Mrs. Jones can be sure of what is expected of her. Moreover, the leader has used imagery to help get the point across. Whenever possible, the leader should use imagery to help participants focus.

Even the arrangement of the room can make a difference in whether participants feel free to join in or not. If the seating is traditional "audience" style, many may not be able to see or hear properly and so are unsure of what is expected. Or those who do want to participate hesitate because it is difficult to come forward. Formal seating suggests "being on stage" and can be inhibiting. All of these difficulties can be eliminated by using a circular seating arrangement. A circle promotes a feeling of closeness from the outset, guarantees that everyone can see equally well and promotes involvement.

The Dominating Participant

The dominating person is easily recognized. He or she talks over everyone else, interrupts, doesn't listen and seems to always insist on being in charge. No matter how exciting a plan you produce, the boss has a better way to do it. He or she wants to make decisions not only for him or herself, but also for everyone else in the group. The boss is often impatient and insensitive to the feelings of others.

What we forget, however, is that this kind of person may behave in such a way because of deep seated insecurities, a lack of trust or a longing for power. On the other hand, this person may have spent many years calling the shots as a leader in industry, education or volunteer work. He or she is accustomed to delegating authority, not sharing it.

There is no question about it, this kind of person can be difficult to deal with. How many times can you hear "I think we ought to . . ." or "There's a better way to do that . . ." or "No, I wouldn't do it that way . . ." in one session without feeling anger well up inside? It's difficult, but becoming defensive will only escalate the confrontation.

Patience, combined with tact, is of the essence when dealing with the boss. "We could go to Mexico by bus, Hattie, but the group just agreed to fly." "Yes, Bill you were excellent as chief of police yesterday, but today it's Jim's turn." A smile is invaluable, this time coupled with a quiet strength that prevents the boss from dominating everyone else in the group.

And then, of course, we can use the boss's ideas but encourage everyone else to elaborate on them so that they become the group's ideas. For example, Phoebe says that she thinks we must plant the garden today. Before she makes all our decisions about seeds, tools, etc., we head her off at the pass. We thank her for her suggestion and quickly ask Margaret whether we should plant flowers or vegetables first. If Phoebe interrupts, we say, "Hold on, Phoebe, let's hear what Margaret has to say."

We can also give the bossy participant responsibility for taking roll, seeing that equipment is ready and in working order, or preparing refreshments. From time to time we can make sure that "the boss" is cast in a leading role or chosen as chairman of a group to satisfy the need for recognition.

Using pair work can also help diminish the power of a boss. If Beverly is working with only one other person, there is less opportunity for her to control the whole group. She is occupied with a partner. If we can pair her with a partner who can stand up to her dominance, all the better.

Counter-attitudinal role playing may also help. In improvisation, the dominant person can be asked to play the role of the newcomer, the weak or helpless one, or the one who is quiet and unsure. Changes are not likely to occur overnight, but a gradual awareness of other modes of behavior can begin to make a difference in the behavior of the boss.

An anecdotal record is useful, both in working with the dominant person and in working with other "difficult to handle" participants. Such a record can help the leader separate behavior from inferences about behavior. Taking a few minutes shortly after each drama session to write down exactly what happened rather than how you feel about what happened can be helpful in planning future sessions. You may, for example, feel that Mrs. Smith is simply impossible to deal with, that she bosses everyone around and makes it so difficult for you to lead the group that you are about to tear your hair out. When you keep an anecdotal record, however, you may find that, in fact, Mrs. Smith only interrupted you two times and told other people in the group what to do only three times. You may discover that, in fact, Mrs. Smith bothers you much more than she bothers the group. You may discover that it is your reaction to Mrs. Smith that really is the problem. She challenges your authority and you find yourself locked in an imagined power struggle with her. Through looking at the situation objectively, via the anecdotal record, you can see that the situation is not as hopeless as you might have thought. You can begin to deal with what is really happening instead of what you infer is happening.

It often comes as a surprise that a personality trait which we find

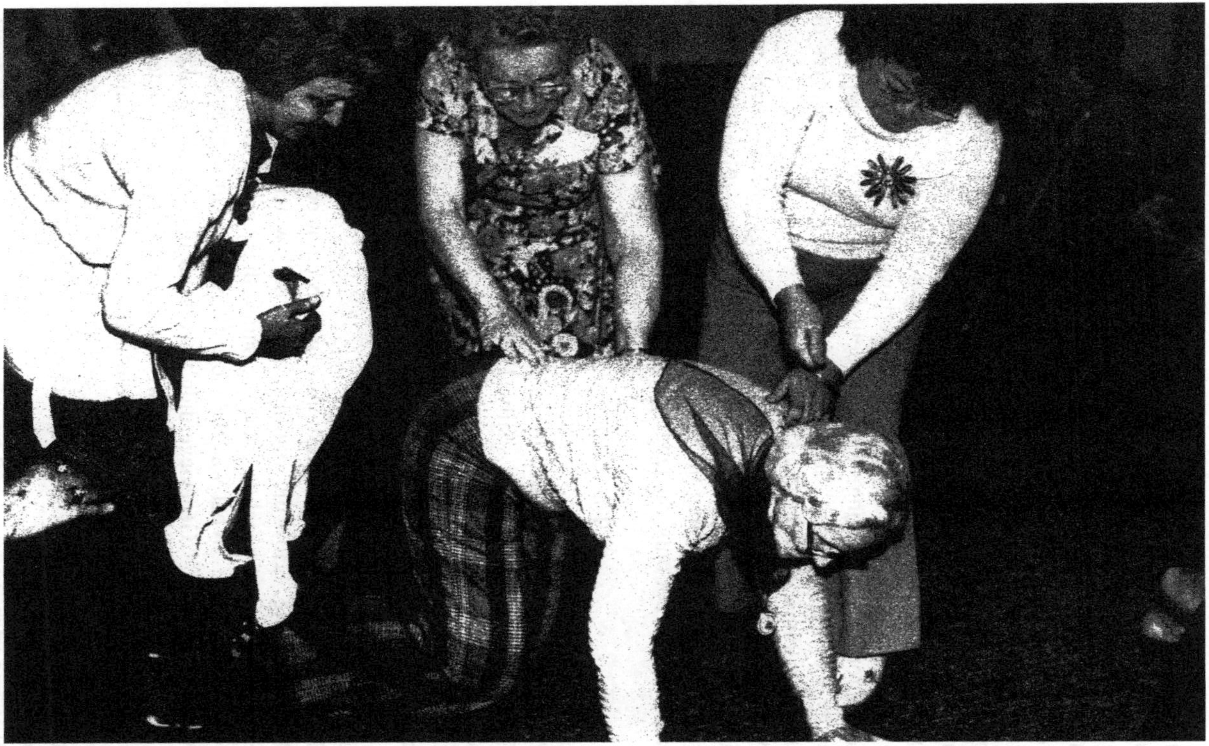

Photo by Dawn Murray

difficult to deal with is not always perceived in the same way by the rest of the group. Perhaps the other participants are so used to Mrs. Smith's bossiness that they no longer pay any attention to it. Or perhaps some of them genuinely appreciate her attention and perceive it as helplessness. Perhaps they have difficulty hearing directions and appreciate her looking out for them. Perhaps some of the more retiring participants depend on the dominant one for leadership. However much we might someday want to see the retiring participants be more independent, they may greatly need whatever support they can get at the beginning. Just as we sometimes encourage participants to get insight into the behavior of others through role playing, we often defuse our hostility or apprehension by viewing "difficult" interpersonal situations through the eyes of participants rather than our own.

We should always remember that the very energy, the life force, that sometimes frustrates us can also become the spark, the driving force for exciting drama. Chanelling the dominating person's initiative and perseverance can be not only challenging but also rewarding.

The Negative Participant

No matter what the leader suggests, the negative participant objects, making comments like, "That's silly. I don't want to stretch right now." When you try an activity or drama game, the critical one denigrates the efforts of others. "Mrs. Brown isn't doing it right," she says, or "I couldn't hear Fred, he never talks loudly enough," or "Genevieve didn't act at all like the ticket taker at the movies." You feel defeated before you start.

But the way you phrase questions can help elicit positive responses. Instead of asking, "How did you like that scene?" which leaves the door open for all kinds of negative criticism, phrase the question to bring forth a positive response: "What was the most interesting part of that scene?" If Mrs. Berres says, "Genevieve didn't act at all like the ticket taker at the movies," you can say, "Oh, but we're talking about the most interesting thing that happened. What did you find most interesting?" You have taken the sting out of the criticism and the steam out of the critic by restating the original question and refusing to be sidetracked by irrelevant criticism.

It is important to avoid getting into a power play in which you insist on trying to turn a negative into a positive comment. "Oh, but Mrs. Berres, surely that wasn't what you meant. You loved the scene, didn't you, Mrs. Berres?" Mrs. Berres probably didn't love the scene (either because it wasn't that good or because she takes pleasure in being very negative) and you are wasting her time, your time and the group's time in what is probably a no-win situation.

If Mrs. Berres is being negative out of a bid for attention, you will probably win her over in the long run by welcoming positive comments and downplaying negative comments. She will soon discover that she will be able to get more attention by contributing positively to the group.

Humor, of course, is one of the best weapons against negativism. Any time we can turn a complaint around and get the complainer laughing with us, we have scored a real victory. This doesn't mean laughing at the complainer, but rather "twisting" their complaint in such a way that they cannot help but see the ridiculousness of it and be amused instead of annoyed. For example, if Art complains that he cannot do the movement exercises today because he is just too tired, we can ask with a twinkle in our eyes, "Oh, Art, are you tired because you were out dancing all night again?" Or when Mildred says she doesn't feel like playing Copy Cat because she'd rather watch, we can say with a smile, "I know, Mildred. You're saving up your energy for that secret admirer of yours. Come on. We know." Such joking comments aren't dwelled on and are made only if we feel the participant will accept and enjoy the humor.

Some people may object that we are not being respectful to the elderly if we kid them, and particularly if we kid them about anything that relates to their sexuality. Indeed some people believe that older adults have neither sexuality nor a sense of humor and that we had better deal with them in a dignified and serious manner, being careful not to offend them. Perhaps.

On the other hand, it is much more likely that senior adults share the full range of human experiences and emotions common to all adults. If we see drama as a way to explore the totality of human experience, if we see drama as a way to reawaken feeling and experience, if we see drama as a joyful, even playful experience, then it seems logical to relate to participants in a fully human way.

Closely related to our attitudes about older adults is the kind of energy level we use when working with them. Many times those who work with the elderly mistakenly believe that they must treat them with kid gloves, as if they were dealing with fragile hot house flowers. They talk softly, move slowly and expect, ask for and get little in response. A high energy level and exciting pace, on the other hand, can make for a much more stimulating environment and can elicit surprising enthusiasm and response. This is especially true when working with someone who is negative. If the leader keeps the pace moving, if the atmosphere is charged with excitement, those who are negative have little time or opportunity to voice complaints. In addition, they may find themselves caught up in the spirit of the session despite their objections. When the leader senses a negative person getting ready for a "tirade," simply picking up the pace of the activity may head the difficulty off at the pass.

The Participant with a Short Attention Span

There are many factors which can cause someone's attention to wander or cause them to turn inward. These range from the physical, such as strokes, post-operational difficulties, depression, medication, low blood pressure, to the emotional, such as feelings of loss caused by the recent death of a loved one or feelings of isolation because of having few ties with family or friends.

Touch is important, as are eye contact and smiles. A gentle touch of the hand or a friendly pat on the shoulder can help participants stay in the here and now or bring them back to the present if they have drifted. Calling a person by name gets attention. "Mrs. James, don't you think this is a beautiful marigold?" A question or brief summary of what's been happening can help promote alertness. "Mrs. James, we're planning what to take along to the beach for our picnic. We're doing a drama about going to the beach. What do you think we ought to pack in our picnic basket?"

Careful pairing of participants for partner work can help too. Those who are more alert can help hold the attention of those who are less alert. Inattentive participants have little opportunity to drift because their partners are speaking or acting directly towards them and expecting a response.

Total group participation is better for the drifter than situations in which one or two people are playing while the others watch or situations which involve long periods of group discussion. For example, if everyone in the group is asked to pantomime looking for a lost ring in the sand, the drifter is encouraged to be doing something and is less likely to sit passively while others talk on and on.

During discussions, it is often helpful to stand next to the person who has difficulty paying attention. This makes it more difficult for that participant to tune you out or drift into a reverie. Your physical proximity is a living reminder that attention is being asked for. In addition, you are insuring that the participant's attention isn't drifting simply because he or she can't hear you.

It will help us if we can remember that there will be different levels of participation for different people. Some will be able to participate fully and joyfully from the beginning. Others will be able to reach a level of joyous participation only with the help and understanding of the leader. Some will always participate minimally because their physical or emotional condition will not allow them to do otherwise.

The Participant with Poor Eyesight

Let us assume that we are dealing here with a person who has lost sight in one or both eyes, who has failing eyesight or is recovering from a cataract operation, but who has reasonably good hearing. The person who can neither see nor hear presents special problems beyond the scope of this book. For the person who has difficulty seeing but who can hear, we must remember to tell ourselves, "ears, ears, ears." In other words, we must remember to continually paint word pictures. Rather than saying, "I brought my grandmother's doll to use in our log cabin drama today," the leader should describe the doll, making it come to life through vivid visual images. "I brought my grandmother's old china doll for us to use in our log cabin drama today. The brown curls are painted so carefully and the cheeks and lips are as red as an apple. I think the eyes are blue glass beads. Perhaps the soft body is stuffed with sawdust. It smells musty. It looks very old. Did any of your grandmothers have a favorite doll?"

In addition to the aural stimuli, touch stimuli should be emphasized. Pass the doll around, being sure the person who has difficulty seeing has the opportunity to explore the doll through touch. When the leader uses a visual stimulus, e.g., a picture, to motivate a session, he or she can describe or ask the group to describe it. In this way those who have difficulty seeing can visualize the content of the picture in their minds. Recorded music, singing and sound effects can be used to stimulate the flow of ideas, particularly for those whose ears are keener than their eyes.

The Participant Who Is Deaf or Hard of Hearing

Let us assume here that we are not dealing with the person who has been deaf all his or her life. This, once again, presents special problems beyond the scope of this book.

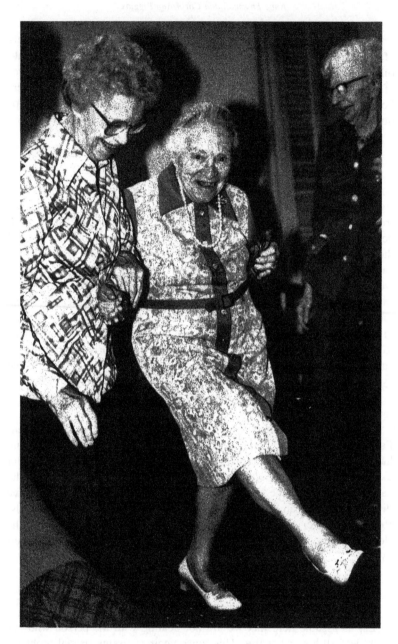

Photo by Dawn Murray

For those who have lost their hearing at an advanced age, there is a continuum stretching from slight hearing impairment to the severely impaired or completely deaf. We often find the person who has difficulty hearing asking us and other participants to repeat over and over again. On the other hand, some are too embarrassed to ask for a repetition and miss or misunderstand directions. The person who cannot hear well often becomes defensive and projects his problem onto others whom he thinks are talking about him or are purposely speaking softly so that he cannot hear.

People who cannot hear well may withdraw from social situations to avoid embarrassment. Those who make an effort to be involved socially may be tense and anxious because they are fearful of missing the thread of conversation or afraid of making mistakes and saying something foolish. Others may alienate the group by continually interrupting conversations with comments that are off the track because they simply haven't heard correctly what has been said.

Hearing aids may be the answer for some, but many people put off either buying or using hearing aids out of pride or for other reasons. Lip reading classes are another possibility but many resist them as well. Even so, there are techniques leaders can use to help the hearing disabled achieve fuller participation. For example, we can repeat the comments of soft-speaking members of the group and stand or sit close to the participant who is having difficulty hearing. We can assign a partner to the hearing disabled to insure that important directions or points of information are understood.

We can be sure to use lots of eye contact and many smiles to reinforce the participant's feeling of welcome and full participation. Touch is important as well as remembering to use the full range of body language in communication. Visual stimulation such as props, pictures, gestures, written instructions, signs and cards, become important.

In a group with many who have difficulty hearing, the leader might want to place heavy emphasis on pantomime and drama that incorporates a good deal of movement. In addition, the use of an aide (another staff member or community volunteer) can also help to guarantee that everyone hears what is going on. Working in pairs is easier than working in groups of five or six, because those who have difficulty hearing can sit closely enough to their partners to hear and to watch lip movements. Leaders should avoid over-enunciating because it causes distortion in the lip reader's interpretation.

Participants Who Are Non-Ambulatory

When we work with participants who are confined to wheelchairs, or must use walkers, casts or crutches, we must obviously adapt many of the drama activities described in this book. On the other hand, leaders must realize that the condition of being non-ambulatory is absolutely no deterrent to a senior adult doing drama. The drama may be more sedentary with greater reliance on dialogue, but there is no reason for it to be exclusively so. Barring medical restrictions, there is no reason for such a participant not to engage in quite a bit of exercise. Rather than protecting the non-ambulatory from movement, we should encourage them to participate to the extent that they are able. The wheelchair bound can move the upper torso. Those with walkers can move about even more, even if the movement is slow.

Physical participation, at first, may be minimal. Muscles that haven't been used for a long time can't be rushed into a flurry of activity. Many seniors have gotten out of the habit of physical exercise and must be encouraged to give it a try. Exercising and energizing through imagery can reduce resistance. For example, if we ask participants to imagine they are lifesize puppets manipulated by a giant puppeteer and then suggest that the strings on various body parts are being lifted and lowered, the motivtion can be so enjoyable that participants forget they are exercising. An instruction such as, "Imagine that you are a soldier puppet saluting the King, then the Queen, then the general of the army," is much more likely to get enthusiastic participation than one like, "Now I want everybody to raise and lower their right arm three times." The first exercise is fun, the second is hard work.

Another way to encourage movement is with music. Participants can play percussion instruments along with recorded music, sway to a rhythmic beat or use hand, arm and upper torso movements while singing. Songs with refrains that everyone knows or action songs with crazy movements are particularly useful. Choice of material is important. Who could resist clicking rhythm sticks to "LaCuccaracha" or shaking a tambourine to "When the Saints Go Marching In."

The non-ambulatory person often has to cope with feelings of uselessness, helplessness, apathy, dependence and being a burden. What better outlet than drama to explore and attempt to come to grips with those feelings. Emotion is central to drama and drama can provide a useful vehicle for the release of feelings. Especially when there are some restrictions on movement, it is important that the dramatic situation be strong

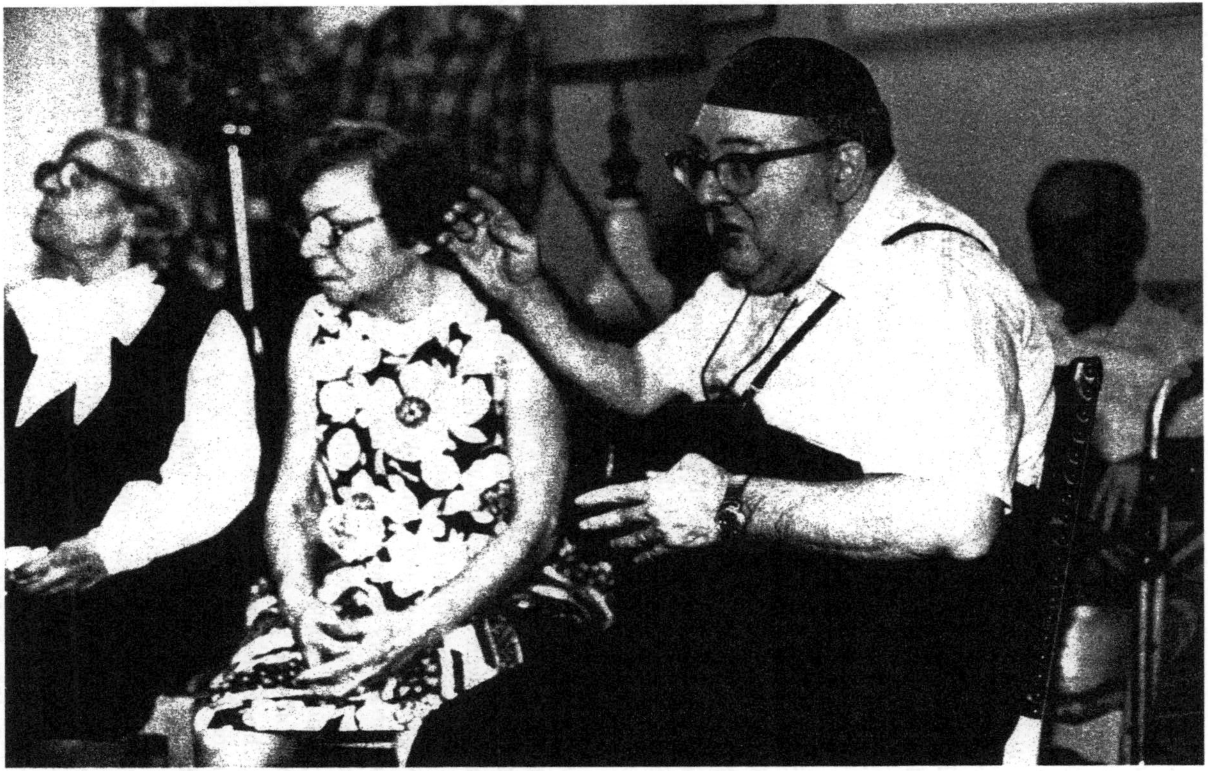

Photo by Dawn Murray

enough to get participants involved. Settings such as an elevator, a restaurant, a mine shaft, an office or a box seat at a football game require limited movement but have dramatic potential. For example, participants may be trapped in an elevator or mine shaft; stage a sit-in at the mayor's office; or find themselves without enough money to pay for their bill at the Waldorf. Non-ambulatory participants, in attacking problems such as these and solving them through dramatic action, can generate an esprit de corps. This can go a long way toward reducing feelings of apathy and helplessness and increasing feelings of self-esteem.

Dealing with Sporadic Attendance

Sporadic attendance can be a problem for the drama leader. Those who attend programs at community centers may be affected by weather conditions, funds for transportation, personal business, part-time jobs or family problems. Of course sporadic attendance can also be a problem in nursing homes. Making sure the drama program is exciting is one of the first solutions to this problem. A drama program that satisfies individual needs, stimulates enjoyment and motivates interaction is essential.

A personal call or note to a frequently absent participant may be all that is needed to bring that participant back to the group. Ask members of the group to remind absentees about the next meeting and to assure them they were missed. If you work in a residential home, you have even greater possibilities for encouraging participation. If you keep the staff abreast of your upcoming plans, they can talk it up and encourage reluctant seniors to join in. An informed nurse's aide may say, "Oh, you don't want to miss drama today, Louise, the group is going to have an auction. People are going to get to keep the things that are auctioned off, and you are even given the money!" Because the aide knows what has been planned, she has a much better chance of talking Louise into coming along.

By the same token, if the drama leader occasionally tells other staff some of the positive things participants have done in previous sessions, the staff may use that information to encourage participation. For example, "I heard what a wonderful job you did playing Twenty Questions, Mr. Johnson. I knew you were clever, but I never knew you were that clever!" Comments that build self-esteem can go a long way in talking Mr. Johnson and others into continuing to come to drama group. The individual feels needed, noticed and admired—feelings we all enjoy.

Dealing with Staff and Administration

Many times the staff and administration are delighted to have a creative drama program going on in their facility. Sometimes, though, there may be problems. Administrators can develop a negative or even hostile attitude toward you and your drama program because of preoccupation with the practical matters of running a home. Staff members may be envious because the drama group is so popular.

To avoid such a situation, be sure everyone knows what creative drama is and what value it has for participants (see Chapter 1). Don't wait for a final evaluation to promote your program with the staff administration. Use a Polaroid camera to take photos of happenings in your group. Not only is it fun and satisfying for participants to see themselves in action, but the photos may be used to design interesting and informative bulletin boards and to document reports. Invite staff members or administrators to help with a session, either in role or by assisting in some other way.

If, despite all your efforts, there still seems to be jealousy and/or hostility, you may have to play down your success and, especially, the "fun" the group is having. It is important to compliment other staff members and administration on their efforts. Some problems can't be solved, some must be accepted and lived with. But it is important to acknowledge that everyone is working in a variety of ways for the well-being of the elderly.

Photo by Dawn Murray

Chapter 5

COMMUNICATING
THROUGH IMPROVISATION

In preceding chapters, materials have been provided to involve seniors in some of the processes most basic to creating drama. But the abilities to pantomime and fully use the senses, for example, while essential to creating good drama, do not in themselves constitute drama. A number of elements must be combined before drama can occur. Chart 1 shows those elements and their relationship to the processes used by players as they create drama.

Elements and Processes of Drama

There are five basic elements in drama: who, what, where, when and why. To have drama, the characters (who) must be involved in solving a problem (what) in a given setting (where) at a particular time (when). A final element is the motivation (why) which explains why a character behaves in a certain way.

The four processes shown in the model—concentration, sensing, thinking and feeling—are the most basic ones involved in creating improvised drama. The drama is expressed and communicated primarily through two modes, movement and speech. Working with the dramatic elements they are given (or choose), players concentrate, use their senses, think and feel to create a spontaneous scene which they share through movement and speech.

Once the participants have experienced a number of predrama games and exercises and have begun to trust their imagination and feel comfortable with each other, they are ready for a more challenging experience. The drama activity can gradually become more complex. Rather than exercising a single dramatic process such as sensing, or a single element such as characterization, participants can now link several elements and processes to create an improvised drama.

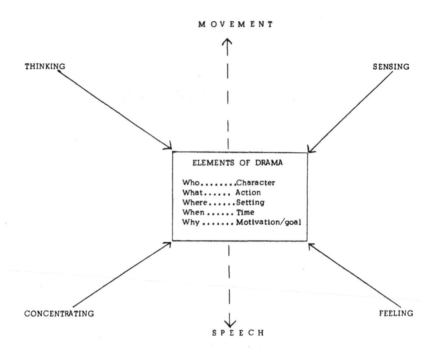

CHART 1: ELEMENTS AND PROCESSES OF IMPROVISED DRAMA

Structuring the Improvisation

We've all heard about the man who was surprised to learn that he had been speaking prose all his life. You may have to remind your seniors that they have been improvising all their lives. They have scolded their children, comforted a sick neighbor or argued with their husbands all without a script.

Although improvisation can be defined as a play (or scene) without a script, that does not mean it starts from nothing. In order for players to create dialogue spontaneously, some information, some structure, must be agreed upon before the scene starts. Usually the given information consists of who is in the scene (characters), where the scene takes place (setting) and what is going on (the initial action or problem).

The dramatic problem, of course, is key to making the improvisation work. Without a problem and the resulting tension, the drama is flat, uninteresting and probably meaningless. The family is leaving on vacation but the car won't start. The family has decided it is time for grandpa to come live with them, but grandpa refuses. Two customers have claimed the last girdle on the half-price table. What will happen? How will the scenes be resolved? Interest is high because the problem demands a solution. The movement toward that solution becomes the dramatic action. Players are now truly doing improvised drama.

At first, the leader needs to provide most of the information, establishing who and where the characters are and the nature of the problem. Participants will be involved primarily in elaborating on the situation and solving the problem. The first improvisations tried by a group are likely to be brief, have sparse dialogue and lack a climax or ending. Although groups may feel more secure in planning every action as well as the ending, this will destroy some of the spontaneity. Encourage the players to trust themselves and allow the ending of a scene to evolve.

Because improvisation provides a more complex structure with greater interaction between characters than many of the drama activities described thus far, increased emotional involvement and a high level of energy will be noted among the players. That energy can infect even the most withdrawn members of the group. Struggling to achieve a goal, to defend one's property, to justify one's position in the face of strong opposition sharpens thinking, intensifies self-belief and results in the release of a torrent of believable dialogue.

It is the leader's responsibility to make sure that the dramatic situation has a problem that is easily understood by the players and piques their interest. In addition, the goals of each character or group of characters must be clear and impelling. It is through trying to reach the goal that the players release the energy needed to make the scene work. In the grandpa's house improv (chart 2), for example, the daughter, grandson and son-in-law want to convince grandpa to move in with them. Grandpa's goal, on the other hand, is to stay right where he is. As the players elaborate they reveal that they are afraid he'll fall down the stairs, that they worry he's not eating right and that they know he's forgetting to take his medicine. Grandpa might counter that he's sleeping in the den now, that Gertrude, the widow across the street, brings him hot meals several times a week and that since he's met her, he doesn't need his medicine any more. His strong desire to maintain his independence, his goal, generates the energy to make the improvisation work.

As the players learn to identify with their roles and work trustingly with each other and to elaborate and play off each other's ideas, the level of belief increases.

Use of limited props and costumes can increase the concentration of

CHART 2: ESTABLISHING DRAMATIC ELEMENTS

WHO (Characters)	WHERE (Setting)	(Initial Situation)	WHAT (Problem)
Family of five	Garage	Loading the car to leave on vacation	The car won't start
Two couples (or)	A field in country posted "No Tres-passing"	On a picnic	A bull suddenly appears
Teacher Father or Mother Teenager	Classroom	Parent-Teacher Conference	Teenager has been cutting class
Dog Catcher Dog's Owner Neighbor	Dogpound	Owner comes to claim dog	Neighbor has filed complaint because dog has destroyed his/her property
Grandpa Daughter Grandson Son-in-law	Grandpa's house	Family has decided it is time for Grandpa to come live with them	Grandpa wants to maintain his independence; is considering remarriage
Boss Employees	Lawnmower factory	Employees have come to complain about safety in factory	Another employee was hurt this week
Teenager Grandma Police	Busy street	Teenager is teaching Grandma to ride a motor scooter	Motor scooter has gone down a one-way street
Doctor Hypochondriac	Clinic	Third check-up in a year for the patient	Doctor can find nothing wrong but patient insists he has several things wrong

the players as well. The use of a stethoscope and tongue depressor for the doctor who is examining the hypochondriac (chart 2) can help both characters believe in their roles.

Groups should not be asked to play scenes for each other until players have gained some self-assurance. It is important to stress that there is no right or wrong way to solve a problem. Any discussion or evaluation of the scenes should stress the positive aspects to help build trust. Criticism must be constructive if the confidence and growth of the players is to be built.

Of any of the drama activities discussed so far, improvisation has the power to take players out of themselves by thrusting them into the immediacy of the scene being played. As players gain more experience, the leader can take a less direct role, with much of the responsibility taken over by participants working in small groups. Flexibility of thought and the ability to "let go" increase as more and more scenes are played and the rediscovery of creative abilities bring pleasure and growing self-confidence to participants.

Improvisational Activities

Following are a number of improvisational activities, some of which are very difficult, others very easy. Some require very little planning, others more. Some spell out the problem, others imply a problem. Some call for the players to determine the problem. In general, easier activities appear first, more challenging ones later.

LIVING PICTURES

Objectives: Work with others in the group to decide on character, setting and problem, but not solution.

Explore how body posture communicates attitudes, feelings and relationships.

Directions: Pictures showing groups of people in different poses and relationships would be helpful, but are not necessary for this activity. A list of situations that suggest living pictures are listed below. Each title can be written on a 3x5 card.

Present one picture or picture title to each group of 4-5 persons. They are to arrange themselves in a still photograph that captures the spirit of the situation. They are to decide where the photograph was taken, what character each is to represent and how they will pose each person in the picture. They should also decide the relationships of the characters to one another. They may talk about anything that has happened before the picture was taken, but are not to plan further than that.

When all plans are made, the leader will ask each group in turn to present its still photo to the rest of the groups. When the leader calls, *Action*, the picture comes to life for a very short time and the characters are to interact as they might in real life. The scene may or may not have an ending. The leader may simply say, *FREEZE IT and thank you*, allowing the players to stop.

The scenes will be rather short and may be done in pantomime the first time the activity is tried. The first time dialogue is used, everyone may talk at once or ideas may emerge slowly. As players find it easier to listen to each other, dialogue will become more spontaneous.

Development: If interest is strong, allow groups time to plan a complete scene.

Subjects For Living Pictures:

The First Baby	Bargain Day at Macy's
Forest Fire*	Three Strikes You're Out*
The Wedding	The Coronation
Auto Accident*	Winner of Million Dollar Lottery

Note: Those subjects marked with an asterisk contain an explicit problem. Others will need to have the problem developed, for example:

The Wedding: the groom loses the ring
the father refuses to give the bride away

The First Baby: baby has bad case of hiccups
                    father and grandmother disagree
                    about the need for fresh air

THE OLD HAT TRICK

Objectives: Communicate through pantomime one aspect of a char-
                  acter, such as occupation.
                  Communicate goal of character being played.
                  Interact with others in solving a problem while planning
                  and playing out a scene.

Directions: This activity requires an assortment of hats which sug-
                  gest character types and occupations. Some can easily
                  be made, others may be found in variety stores and
                  rummage sales.

                  Holding up one hat at a time, the leader may ask such
                  questions as:

                  1. *What can you tell me about the person who wears
                     this hat?*
                  2. *Would you say he or she is neat or sloppy?*
                  3. *Do you think the person is lazy? Energetic?
                     Lucky? Proud? Shy? Intelligent? Generous?*
                  4. *What does this person look forward to each day?*

                  Ask the group to show in pantomime something this
                  person would do on an ordinary work day. Then share
                  their ideas verbally. Although they will be working with
                  the same hat as a stimulus, their ideas will be diverse.
                  This diversity should be fully noted during the discus-
                  sion following the activity.

Development: After the group has created occupations and actions for
                  several characters, they may want to share their panto-
                  mimes one at a time, or they may be ready to add
                  dialogue and create a short improvisation. Arrange hats
                  into groups of three. For each group provide: 1) a place
                  for the scene to take place; and 2) a problem for the

characters to work on. Give each group 5-10 minutes to discuss their ideas, then share the scenes.

The following information is written on cards and given to the various groups.

#1　Where: Throne Roome
　　Characters: King, Maid, Clown
　　Problem: Maid is trying to get a date with clown

#2　Where: Deep Woods
　　Characters: Baker, Witch, Baby
　　Problem: Baker wants to get a recipe from the
　　　　　　 witch

#3　Where: Outside a barn
　　Characters: Farmer, Nurse, Robin Hood
　　Problem: Robin Hood needs first aid

#4　Where: Indian Reservation
　　Characters: Indian, Cowboy, Engineer
　　Problem: Cowboy looking for lost bull

#5　Where: Alaska
　　Characters: Eskimo, Soldier. Motorcyclist
　　Problem: Soldier must evict Eskimo to build
　　　　　　 airstrip

Ideas for the Hat Collection

King (crown)	Farmer (straw hat)
Maid (frilly cap)	Robin Hood (green/feather)
Clown (pointed hat)	Nurse (white/stiff)
Baker (puffed top)	Cowboy (ten gallon)
Witch (pointed hat)	Engineer (striped cap)
Baby (bonnet)	Indian (feathers on band)
Cyclist (crash helmet)	Eskimo (fur hood)
Fireman (red helmet)	Mexican (sombrero)
Uppercrust (derby)	Hunter (red hat)

Discussion:　Questions such as the following can be asked after the playing of each scene:

1. *How did the players let us know where the scene was taking place?*
2. *Would you have known who the characters were even if they hadn't been wearing hats? What other cues did they give us?*
3. *How did the players make it believable that three such different characters were in the same place?*
4. *Were you surprised at the way they solved the problem? What made the solution unusual? Amusing? Fitting?*

PROVERBS

Objectives: Improvise a situation which embodies the truth and spirit of a chosen proverb.

Develop creative thinking, particularly the ability to elaborate and work by analogy.

Materials: A list of proverbs:

1. Birds of a feather flock together.
2. Nothing ventured, nothing gained.
3. Let sleeping dogs lie.
4. Half a loaf is better than none.
5. Every cloud has a silver lining.
6. Haste makes waste.
7. It is never too late to learn.
8. Don't count your chickens before they're hatched.
9. Actions speak louder than words.
10. Too many cooks spoil the broth.
11. A new broom sweeps clean.
12. Two heads are better than one.
13. A bird in the hand is worth two in the bush.
14. Absence makes the heart grow fonder.

Activities: Ask members of the group to share proverbs they heard as a child. Select one and discuss what it really means and how it could apply in several ways of situations. For example, "Every cloud has a silver lining," is not really about clouds but is a metaphor indicating that good luck follows bad, happiness follows pain. Discuss real or imaginary situations that might bear this proverb out.

Leader guides group to plan an improvisation based on a single proverb. Or, small groups can plan and enact a scene. Each group may be given the same proverb or each may be given a different one.

RAISING A FAMILY

Objectives: Explore similarities and differences in the practice of raising children.
Compare past and present methods of child rearing.

Materials: Sign "Spare the Rod and Spoil the Child"

Activities: Discuss this adage in terms of how members of the group were raised. Did they raise their children according to the same or different principles? Were there any disagreements between mother and father, husband and wife concerning the ways children should be raised?

Have group list some of the most troublesome problems in child rearing and some of the approaches and solutions that were tried.

Development: Improvise scenes based on successful and unsuccessful approaches.

Discussion: Discuss how some children are raised differently today.

DOWN MEMORY LANE #2

Objectives: Share memories about a particular time in life.
Carry out one person's memory in an improvisation.
Take initiative and show responsibility for the planning
and playing of the scene.

Directions: Write on a blackboard or large sheet of paper the following:
> Home Memories
> Grade School Memories
> High School Memories
> College Memories
> First Job Memories

Play a recording of "Memories," or sing the song. Discuss which of the above types of memories are strong-
est. Funniest. Strangest.

Ask participants to choose which group of memories
they are most interested in. Try to allow no more than
five in each group. If there is no interest in a certain
category, or if there are enough players to make two
groups in one category, do not be concerned. Each
scene will turn out quite differently.

Give each group the accompanying list of questions to
start their discussions. These are meant as starters only.
Allow 10-15 minutes for this preliminary discussion.
Assure participants that they are not to be limited by
these questions.

At the end of 15 minutes, ask that each group select
one experience to serve as the basis of their improvisation. Then they must decide:

> WHERE   the scene takes place
> WHO   are the characters in the scene
> WHAT   happens in the scene; who has a prob-
> lem and how does it work out

After another 5-10 minutes of planning in groups, the
scenes should be shared.

DISCUSSION QUESTIONS FOR SMALL GROUPS

Home Memories

1. *What were some of the problems or troubles you had with family pets?*
2. *What was your favorite family vacation?*
3. *What did you and your brothers/sisters fight about?*
4. *Can you remember some surprises that happened on your birthday?*
5. *What traditions did your family observe that were important to you?*

Grammar School Memories

1. *What do you remember about your first day at school?*
2. *How did you meet your best friend?*
3. *What was the most embarrassing day at school?*
4. *What pranks did you play on your classmates?*
5. *Was there a school comedian? What do you remember about him/her?*

High School Memories

1. *What can you remember about your first date?*
2. *What was your after school job?*
3. *What clubs or after school activities did you participate in?*
4. *What was your favorite class and why?*
5. *What styles were popular when you went to high school? How did your mother feel about the "newer" styles?*

College Memories

1. *Are there any funny/interesting stories about you and your roommates?*
2. *What were the high-jinks or jokes that were carried on by the fraternity boys?*
3. *Did you have any attitude changes during the college years? Such as?*
4. *What songs were popular when you were in college?*
5. *Did your school have a campus hangout? What went on there?*

First Job Memories

1. *What was your first job and how did you get it? Do you remember your salary?*
2. *Can you remember how you spent your first check?*
3. *What was your first day on the job like?*
4. *What do you think you learned in your first job that has helped you in your life?*
5. *What funny or scary things happened during your first job?*

Note: Any one of these twenty situations could be the basis for a complete session of drama allowing several groups to share their interpretation of the same kind of memory.

SCANDALS

Objectives: Recall details of notorious events and translate them into action.

Compare scandals of the past with the present.

Materials: Signs simulating newspaper headlines posted around the room to attract attention and start discussion.

Tea Pot Dome Boils Over
Ingrid Bergman has Love Child
Edward VIII Abdicates for Wallis Simpson
White Sox Win Pennant

Activities: Share memories of events evoked by the signs. Draw out details of other scandals remembered by the group. Choose one or two of these to use as the basis of an improvisation. The event itself may not be at the center of the improvisation, but rather the reaction of others to the event. Repeat process with more contemporary scandals.

Discussion: *Why did this event cause such concern? Have there been similar events in the past few years? Would the*

*public react today as it did at the time of the scandal?
Are today's scandals of a different type than those thirty
years ago?*

SAFETY ON THE STREETS

Objectives: Articulate concerns relating to safety.
Propose some solutions to problems of safety for seniors.

Materials: Newspaper clipping of a mugging or related safety
problem facing elderly people.
Simulated microphone for Man on the Street.
Sign: "Safety on the Streets for Senior Citizens."

Activity: Leader takes the role of interviewer on the "Man on the
Street Program." Leader announces the topic for the
day, "Safety on the Streets for Senior Citizens" and the
location of the broadcast. The leader welcomes those in
the audience and thanks them for coming and being willing to answer some questions. With each person called
on, a few personal questions may be asked before
getting to the subject at hand.

Possible questions:

1. *Is the situation on the streets at night a lot worse
   today than a decade ago? In what way, would you
   say?*
2. *Do you think newspaper and TV reports exag-
   gerate the situation?*
3. *Do you think it would be better if such incidents
   were kept out of the news?*
4. *What do you think are the causes of the seeming
   increase in attacks?*
5. *What is being done to remedy the situation? What
   could be done?*
6. *What can seniors themselves do to help?*
7. *Could seniors help by working with schools?
   neighborhood groups? the police? mayor's office?*

Development: Set up improvisations based on some of the positive constructive suggestions. Worthy ideas might be passed along to the proper authorities.

AMALGAMATED OBJECTS, LTD.

Objectives: Develop teamwork in a problem solving activity.
Display creativity in relating seemingly unrelated objects.
React spontaneously while in role.

Directions: The leader holds up three objects, one at a time, asking that they first be identified and then asking for any comments about each object's uniqueness. The leader then explains that participants will use these objects to suggest basic elements for a scene. For example:

A. One object should suggest *where* the scene takes place.
B. One object should suggest a *problem* for the scene.
C. One object should suggest a *solution* to the problem.

Decide with the group which object is to be used for each of the above elements. For example:

A. Paperweight = where = (office)
B. Agatha Christie novel = problem = (secretary is caught reading on job)
C. Vase = solution = (flowers for boss and promise to read mysteries at home)
D. Characters: boss, secretary, delivery boy who brings flowers, clerk from next door

Groups of four are given three objects and time to plan their scenes. The leader will circulate among the groups to make sure they have decided on the function of each object.

The playing of scenes will generate a lot of fun, especially as players go beyond their original plans and spontaneously react to other players as well as audience.

Some objects that might be used are:

Candlestick	Driver's license	Handcuffs
Sheriff's badge	Razor	Briefcase
Murder Mystery	Pillow	Garden trowel
Knife	Typewriter	Can of dog food
Tennis racquet	Vase	Matches
Wine skin	Coffeepot	Deck of cards
Recording	Scissors	Bank statement
Calculator	Beer can	Birthday card
Doll	Paperweight	Xmas tree ornament
Cook book	Curling iron	Billfold
Theatre ticket	TV guide	Sheet
Toy		

GREAT BEGINNINGS

Objectives: Develop problem-solving and decision-making skills. Communicate response to an imaginary environment. Create spontaneous dialogue; learn to give and take in scene playing.

Directions: Divide participants into groups of 4 or 5. Each group is given a sentence typed on a card. That sentence must be the very first thing said in an improvised scene.

The leader gives time for groups to plan. They must decide where the scene takes place, who the characters are and who speaks the given sentence but are not to plan how the scene ends. Groups may or may not be able to bring the scene to a conclusion, depending upon the amount of experience they have had in scene playing. The leader asks each group to form a tableau to form a point of departure for its scene.

Examples of sentences that might be used are as follows:

The lion just got loose!
We're lost!
How long will the oxygen hold out?
I smell smoke!
I'm afraid of heights!
The car won't start!
I dare you!
Jean is missing!
Where's the plutonium?
I said you're all fired . . . and that's that!
Orange, orange, I tell you it's got to be orange!
Surprise!
Call the ambulance!
Shall we shoot him now or later?

GREAT ENDINGS

Objectives: Plan a scene with a beginning and middle which leads
logically to the last line.

Initiate ideas and share with others in the planning and
playing of a scene.

Develop fluency and assurance in spontaneous action
and dialogue.

Directions: This scene is more difficult than Great Beginnings and
may require more help from the leader.

Divide participants into groups of 4-5. Each group is
given a sentence typed on a card. The group is to plan
a scene using the given sentence as the last words said
in the scene.

Groups must decide who they are, where the scene
takes place, what problem they are having and how it
will be resolved. Ask them to start the scene in a still
photograph.

Examples of sentence/phrases that might be used are as
follows:

I found the key!
I'm never going to listen to you again!
No one's going to believe this!
This is going to make headlines!
I never believed in flying saucers before!
And the authorities closed it down!
Let's call it a night!
The fire is out!
Oh, no, not another one!
Thank goodness the elephant is sedated!

Improvisation Starters

The leader is encouraged to create improvisations that are tailored to his or her particular group. After deciding who is in the scene and where the scene takes place, the leader chooses a problem which will involve all the characters. The scene could involve three circus performers trying to convince the owner of the circus not to close the show or a gold prospector and a cowboy being fleeced by a card shark in the saloon. A list of characters and settings is included here to aid the leader in constructing improvisations.

LIST OF SETTINGS (WHERE) FOR DRAMA

cave	lobby	pet shop
moon	subway station	social worker's office
doctor's waiting room	restaurant	flower garden
elevator	wharf	ice skating rink
wax museum	trading post	ballpark
carnival	market place	real estate office
toy factory	beach	retirement home
alley in a big city	kitchen	bus station
forest	haunted house	post office
jungle	basement	movie theatre
race track	city park	museum
wagon train	grocery store	historical society
dog show	dentist's office	city hall
airport	art gallery	church/parish hall
bakery	backstage	police station
campsite	shipwrecked	driving license bureau

desert	amusement park	bar/tavern
ship	circus	supermarket
palace	classroom	radio/TV station
busy street corner	hospital	rummage sale
lost/found department	zoo	state fair
attic	family gathering	airplane
apartment	barnyard	clock shop
concert	farm	garage
gymnasium	hotel lobby	hotel room
lakeside in winter	laundromat	library
site of an accident	lighthouse	

LIST OF CHARACTERS (WHO) FOR DRAMA

bus driver	zookeeper	mothers
teacher	dentist	fathers
fireman	baseball player	grandpas
policeman	shoe clerk	grandmas
street cleaner	beautician	balloon man
sailor	horseback rider	Santa Claus
soldier	principal	magicians
pilgrim	boy/girl scout leader	hunters
cowboy	gym teacher	lion tamer
shepherd	plumber	weightlifter
princess	pizza maker	tight rope walker
prince	scientist	train engineer
milkman	robot	race car driver
mailman	elevator operator	airplane stewardess
doctor	sculptor	pilot
nurse	gold prospector	farmer
garbage man	tennis player	clown
ice cream man	TV repairman	ballerina
janitor	Eskimo	baker
king	inventor	deepsea fisherman
queen	detective	babysitter
astronaut	lifeguard	cartoon characters
ice skater	truck driver	snake charmer
carpenter	bus driver	parachutist
gardener	mermaids	famous inventor
secretary	toy maker	prisoner

barber	wild animals	frontiersman
cashier	domestic animals	film maker
salesman	devil	glassblower
forest ranger	juggler	oceanographer
news reporter	ringmaster	geologist
judge	bricklayer	jeweler
astronaut	cook	interior designer
cobbler	jogger	politician
weatherman	tour guide	monk
dancer	lawyer	author
home economics teacher	basketball player	lifeguard
truant officer	actress	social worker
radio announcer	spy	landlord
witch	ambulance driver	sewer worker
ghost	model	used car salesman
flower seller	gambler	mountain climber
painter	bank teller	auto mechanic
grocery clerk	waitress	junk dealer
bull fighter	fortune teller	auctioneer
President	short order cook	army sergeant
football player	telephone operator	rag & bone man
tourists	tailor/seamstress	rock singer
historic figure	cheerleader	computer operator
gangsters	taxi driver	hermit
millionaire	bell boy	photographer
fashion merchandiser	spoiled child	movie star
architect	political agitator	bum/hobo
migrant harvester	strikers	missionary
prisoner of war	skyjacker	beggar
jury member	lion hunter	coal miner
brain surgeon	smuggler	slave
new immigrant	gypsy fortune teller	athletic coach
conservationist	museum curator	prize fighter/wrestler
karate expert	Biblical characters	band leader
mind reader	veterinarian	jockey
pioneer	stock market broker	construction worker
archeologist	runaways	World War I aviator
future planners	Priest/Rabbi/Nun	minister
returning war victim	skier	gunsmith
jet set traveler	electrician	ship's captain

gang members	frogman	librarian
pool shark	horse trainers	mayor
secret agents	disk jockey	cavemen
concert pianist	Olympic champion	carnival barker
newsboy		

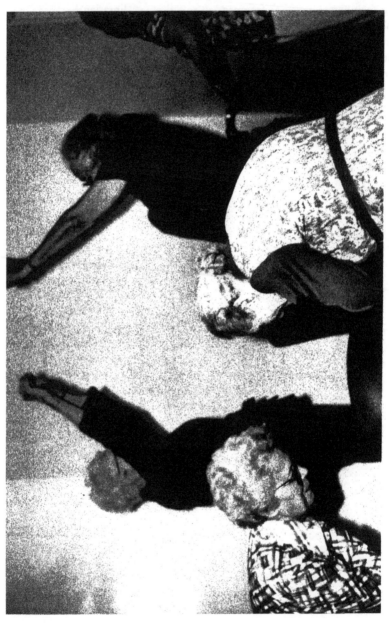

Photo by Dawn Murray

Chapter 6

PLANNING A SESSION
WITH A UNIFYING THEME

Once interest in creative drama has been sparked and confidence has grown through participation in pre-drama exercises, drama games and improvisation, the group is ready to embark on a deeper, more meaningful experience. This can be provided by organizing the drama session around a unifying theme.

If all the activities of a session are related to the theme, for example, of friendship or of Thanksgiving or gardening, the impact of each activity can be increased. The entire drama session becomes more memorable, transitions from one activity to another can be made more smoothly, associations flow more freely and a greater sense of closure can be achieved. The use of a unifying theme provides dramatic focus and eliminates fragmentation. Exploring a theme like friendship through warm-ups, songs, pantomime, sharing of memories, improvisation and discussion allows for sharing a many-faceted view which illuminates and extends our notion of what it is to be human. The whole experience becomes greater than the sum of the parts.

Selecting a Theme

Leaders get ideas from many sources. Themes may come from books or films or TV programs. They may come from something that happened on a shopping trip or visit to the zoo. Holidays, vacations or hobbies may stimulate ideas just as pet peeves, surprises or accidents do. Other sources for ideas might be pets; newspaper articles; diary entries; pictures or cartoons; family, relatives or friends; or the drama group itself. In short, the entire web of human experience may yield ideas for the theme of a drama session.

For example, take Mary Peterson, an activity director at a residential care facility, who is trying to plan her vacation. As a first step, she goes to see her travel agent. While waiting for her appointment, she glances around the office at the travel posters and is struck by the colorfulness of the poster of Mexican folk dancers. "What a good idea," she thinks to herself, "for the focus of a drama session or two." Mary quickly jots her idea down in a notebook she carries expressly for the purpose of holding on to those brainstorms she has. She has no time to develop the idea now, but she doesn't want to lose it.

Brainstorming for Images

Later, when Mary begins to plan the session, she will brainstorm on paper. She will write down as many images as she can that relate to the concept of a Mexican vacation. There is complete freedom of association at this point. Any idea is all right. Selection will come later. Mary writes down the following:

bullfight	cliff divers	pinata
picador	Popocatepetl	hot sun
matador	jumping beans	bright colors
bull	silver	pesos
sombrero	tin	open air markets
wetbacks	castinets	maracas
floating flower gardens	churches	guitar
border guards	margaritas	refried beans
colorful costumes	hat dance	tostados
adobe	enchiladas	El Mexico (airline)

Selecting and Sequencing the Activities

Mary then selects those aspects of the theme that she thinks will be most appealing to the particular group with whom she works and that will, at the same time, offer the most dramatic possibilities. Which images will provide the opportunity for movement and characterization? For conflict and dramatic tension? Which will provide the greatest opportunity for interaction? Mary limits her selection to no more than three or four main images. She then groups other images which relate to and support each main image.

MAIN IMAGES	RELATED ACTIVITIES
Airline El Mexico	buying tickets packing a suitcase eating meal on the plane creating an in-flight talent show taking roles of crew
Bullfight	reacting to hot sun, bright colors vendors hawking refreshments cheering the picador and matador moving as the bull; attacking, feinting
Open Air Market	bargaining with sellers of maracas, castanets, pottery, etc. trying on serape, sombreros, shawls, etc. tasting tacos and other food becoming vendors demonstrating and describing their wares

The Need for Objectives

Mary needs to determine beforehand what the objectives of the session will be. What does she hope participants will do, say or experience? Identifying goals beforehand helps to insure that there is some depth, some purpose to each experience she chooses.

Mary commits her objectives and the rest of her plan to paper to help clarify the progression of the session in her mind. For her Mexican drama, Mary chooses the following objectives for her participants:

1. Recall experiences related to travel, vacations or Mexico.
2. Use previously known and new information (travel folders) in decision making.
3. Decide clothing and personal needs appropriate to the trip to be taken and pantomime packing.
4. Work together, responding spontaneously to each other and to several environments.

In general, it is helpful if objectives are stated in terms of the hoped for behavior of participants. It is easier to observe behavior than to observe feelings or thoughts. "Participants will verbally recall memories of their childhood," is a much easier objective than, "Participants will feel comfortable in the group." The willingness of participants to share their memories may well indicate they are feeling comfortable, but we can only observe the behavior, not the attitudes or emotions that prompt it.

Objectives serve as a guide for the selection of appropriate activities. In addition, they help to keep the leader "on track" during the drama session by providing guidelines for questioning and interaction with the group. After the session, the objectives become the criteria for evaluating the involvement of participants and the success of the leader.

So far Mary has decided on the theme for her drama session, has brainstormed images, selected activities and determined the objectives she hopes will be evidenced by the participants. Now she must plan how to introduce the idea of a Mexican vacation to her group. How will she use the travel poster? Will she use some Mexican music? A costume?

Planning the Introduction

Mary considers materials and motivation carefully as she decides how to introduce her Mexican vacation session. She chooses stimulus objects and questions that will spark the group's interest in taking a trip to Mexico. Whatever objects and/or questions she chooses must do several things for her. They must quickly communicate the general theme. They must evoke associations that relate to the concept whether experienced directly or through films, books or in some other way. In addition, the stimulus objects and questions can help to reveal the feelings of participants about Mexico and indicate which aspects of the country they find most interesting.

Mary plans to tape posters of Mexico around the drama room so participants will see them as soon as they enter. She decides to wear brightly colored clothes evocative of Mexico such as a colorful skirt, or a shawl, cape, bolero, sombrero, or serape to further arrest the attention of the group. She might plan to pass out a tostito to each participant to munch on during the introduction to the session as she greets them in Spanish, "Hola! Buenos Dias, Amigos. Como esta ustedes?" She may plan then to drop her Spanish accent and speak in her own voice, asking a question such as, "Why do you think so many people seem to go to Mexico for vacation?" The use of open-ended questions, those providing opportunities for an unlimited number of appropriate responses, is the most crucial strategy for the leader to master. When phrased carefully, open-ended questions can help to overcome inertia, generate enthusiasm and lead participants to active involvement.

Planning the Development

Mary recognizes that props can be useful in focusing attention and in drawing participants into the drama. She plans to distribute travel folders of Mexico. As each participant accepts her colorful offering, they will have taken the first step into pretense. When she announces that the group has won a free trip to Mexico, participants will be more willing to go along with her "big lie" because the travel folders have provided a bridge from reality into the realm of imagination. Once they have crossed over this bridge to the "as if" world, they become committed to the drama.

Mary knows that this agreement to pretense will be difficult for some participants, but she also knows that her own willingness to suspend disbelief is crucial to gaining the commitment of most participants. She must be absolutely convincing when she announces that the group has won a trip. Her excitement and enthusiasm calls forth excitement and enthusiasm from the group.

Now she must be armed with a battery of questions to sustain and deepen the belief. "Where in Mexico would you like to go? What things could we do in Mexico City? What time of year shall we go? Shall we stay in Mexico City or shall we travel around the countryside?" The first two questions will draw out all relevant information about Mexico and help Mary see where she needs to feed in further information. These questions also help her to ascertain the level of enthusiasm in the group. Allowing participants to make a choice as to the time of year assures them that this is their drama. Their decisions count. As participants defend their preferences to stay in Mexico City or visit the countryside, tremendous energy is released and commitment to the dramatic pretense is strengthened.

As a next step in helping participants identify with the dramatic situation, Mary plans to involve the group in role playing. She will choose a volunteer to sell tickets at the airlines office while she takes the role of the tour leader. At this point, no other individual characters have been delineated. Only a group identity has been established. Risk is low but excitement is missing. Unless group members introduce it themselves, there is no conflict, there are no problems, there is no tension.

Mary knows that in her role of tour leader, she can introduce tension and provide clues for character differentiation. Of course there are many ways of going about this. She may directly challenge some of the tour group members. "I'm sorry, Fred. You can't possibly bring your St. Bernard along." She can get a call on an imaginary telephone informing her that all members of the tour must have a shot to protect them from a recent outbreak of typhus in Acapulco. She could ask participants to suggest things that might go wrong in the ticket office or might slow down the purchase process. Or she could introduce tension by providing selected participants with problem cards. One of these cards might read, "You have a phobia about flying and want to inspect the plane before you buy your ticket." Another card might read, "You insist on taking your parakeet Hercules with you."

To provide more physical action, Mary plans to have participants pantomime packing their bags in preparation for the trip. She will encourage them to pack clothes they have always wanted or have imagined themselves wearing, rather than packing only clothes they presently own. To help them visualize the items they're packing, she will give verbal clues like, "Does anyone need tissue paper to keep your clothes from mussing? I have some spot remover if anyone needs it. Don't forget a sweater or jacket. It gets chilly at night. What might you take on this trip that nobody else in this room might think of? Something really special or unusual." She will also enter into the "as if" situation by "collecting" unused hangers and "checking" the locks on bags so that she can help to sustain belief. Although she knows that the actual pantomime might last no longer than 60 seconds, she recognizes that it can generate much animated discussion about what each participant selected and why.

At this point in her planning, Mary realizes that she has much more material than she will need for one session so she decides to spend several days on the Mexican drama. The plane trip, bull fight and market place will have to wait for a second and third day. Before planning those sessions, though, she needs to plan a wrap up for the first session, reviewing what has happened and relating it to participants' lives.

Concluding the Session

It is important for Mary to allow five to ten minutes at the end of the session for members to share their feelings and reactions about the drama. She knows that participating in the drama is not enough. Members should be led to see the relationship of the drama to their own lives and the lives of others and to discover a personal meaning within the drama.

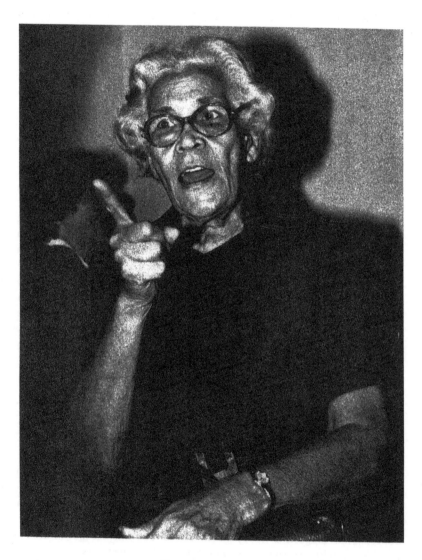

Photo by Dawn Murray

To get the ball rolling, she might ask for group response to several questions, e.g., "How many people brought their bathing suits? Did anybody bring a camera or tape recorder? Did anyone pack an umbrella? Sunglasses?" She really doesn't care how many people answer yes or no or who has just now decided they should have packed a camera. She is primarily building enthusiasm for the trip and encouraging people to respond. Because answering the questions requires only a show of hands, there is little risk for participants as they respond.

Next she will ask more open-ended questions which will require individual responses rather than a show of hands. "Would someone share with us what you packed for evening wear? A day in the mountains? Shopping in Mexico City?" The questions will be phrased in such a way to focus the response. Mary will seek answers from several people, commenting on likenesses and differences. Mary realizes that talking about and describing the objects that have been packed helps make them and hence the trip more real. She can help participants visualize each item in even greater detail by "seeing" the object herself and elaborating on each individual's contribution. If Mrs. Peterson says she is going to take her diamond tiara for evening wear, Mary may say, "Oh, is that the one you wore at the Christmas party last year? The one with the sapphire? How much do you have it insured for?"

Now she will relate back to a question she asked during the packing scene. "What was the one special or unusual thing you packed? The thing that nobody else in the room might have thought of?" The very wording of the question is a subtle press to go beyond the usual, the conventional, the first idea that pops into your head. The word "unusual" makes us search for something unique. This will also give Mary the opportunity to build the self-image of participants by honoring unique responses. When Fred says, "I packed my hot water bottle," Mary can say, "What a good idea. I never thought of that. We'll all borrow it when our backs ache after our backpacking outing."

When Felicia says she packed her butterfly net, Mary will be given the opportunity to individualize another character for the group's drama. Butterfly net suggests a hobby which carries one into the out-of-doors. To Mary, it will also suggest a careful person, a patient person, a person with a strong response to nature, to color, to the environment. The trip to Mexico will afford Felicia the opportunity to collect specimens she has never seen before. Because Mary sees these possibilities, she can help Felicia see them. When Felicia bought her ticket at the beginning of the drama session, she was just another member of the tour. But now she is beginning to be a distinct character with a character-related goal for going on the trip.

Finally, Mary plans to relate what has happened in the drama session to the lives of participants. Through a summary discussion, she will help them discover a personal meaning in the experience. There are many themes explicitly or implicitly imbedded in this session. The whole idea of winning, for example, or decision making and consensus, travel, vacations or the tyranny of the airline computer. Obviously, the session involves arrival at consensus concerning when and where and what in Mexico, and individual decisions in the packing. But because she cannot predict the degree of resistance or avoidance to the theme of decision making, she chooses to go with vacations because it's safer. Most of her people have been on a vacation of some sort or another. Whether at a cottage, an automobile trip, or a visit to relatives in Europe, or simply staying at home, the concept is a familiar one and bound to elicit a flow of ideas.

Because she wants the group to explore the common denominators of their thought and experience as well as the infinite variety it can assume, she plans to lead them to reflect on the reasons and purposes for vacations. Are vacations for excitement, adventure, fulfillment? Are they for refreshment, rest, introspection? She will ask them to consider why different people choose different kinds of vacations. She will deepen the exploration by knitting together what participants have experienced in the drama with what they have experienced in their past lives. Questions like the following will help:

1. Of any of the vacations you took as a child, which do you remember most vividly?
2. Did anything unexpected ever happen to you or your family on a vacation?
3. Was there one day or one time when your family felt closest together on a vacation?
4. How and by whom were family vacations planned?
5. What was the funniest thing that ever happened on a vacation?

Keeping in mind that Mary has planned this as one of several sessions on a Mexican vacation (full plan following), many other themes will be explored in the second, third and fourth days. For example, "The Bullfight" may suggest the theme of hunter and hunted or spectator sports.

Tempting though it is to allow the drama to absorb the entire session,

Mary knows that assuring time for reflection is essential. Exciting though the dramatic enactment may be, it is only through the discovery of its significance for each participant that it reaches its full potential to touch and transform lives.

MEXICAN VACATION

Objectives:

1. Recall experiences related to travel, vacations or Mexico.

2. Use previously known and new information (travel folders) in decision making.

3. Decide clothing and personal needs appropriate to the trip to be taken and pantomime packing.

4. Work together, responding spontaneously to each other and to several environments.

5. Communicate through pantomime and verbal description imaginary objects found in the market place.

6. Interact (spiritedly) in pairs as shoppers and vendors each attempting to reach a goal.

Before the Session:

1. Try to find travel posters of Mexico or colorful pictures from magazines.

2. Assemble materials:

   a. Mariachi music (from the library)

   b. sombrero, serape

   c. tostados

   d. pinata if possible (if you do not have access to one, substitute a brightly painted paper bag filled with wrapped candies, etc.)

   e. maracas or gourds with dried seeds (if you do not have access to either, try taping two paper cups together after putting five or ten dried beans in one. The cups may be brightly painted if you wish.)

f. airline travel folders about Mexico

3. The leader might wish to dress with a brightly colored skirt or shirt and, for a woman, large hoop earrings.

Introduction: 1. Greet each participant as he or she arrives. Make a personal comment to each or ask a question of each.

2. Play mariachi music and pass out tostitos to participants to munch on.

3. Leader may want to call out a few ole's and other Spanish phrases.

Development: *Planning the trip*

1. With participants seated in a circle, distribute travel folders. Explain that the group has won a free trip to Mexico and will have to decide where to go.

2. "Which parts of Mexico would you like to see? Mountains? Seaside? Mexico City?" "What is it about Mexico City that makes you think we should visit there?" or "If we visited Mexico City, what things could we do there?" or "What time of year shall we go?" or "Shall we stay in Mexico City or should we travel around the countryside a bit?"

3. After some discussion, try to bring the group to a consensus or vote on your destination.

4. Explain that since we've won the tickets as a prize, we won't have to pay for them, but that we will have to go down to the airline ticket office to pick them up. Ask for a volunteer to be the clerk at the ticket office. Leader may want to act as the tour director to help things along. Improvise the group going to the ticket office to pick up their tickets. Perhaps each participant could be given a number at

the office, so that the ticket agent can simply call
out the next client to pick up their tickets. Some
complications could arise to make the scene more
interesting. (These could be discussed beforehand
or printed on small 3x5 cards given to each participant.)

a. You have a phobia about flying and insist on
inspecting the plane before you buy your ticket.

b. You insist on taking your parakeet Hercules with
you and will not allow him to be placed in the
baggage compartment.

c. You get airsick very easily and are concerned
about the amount of turbulence.

d. You want a seat over the wing and are distressed
when the ticket agent says no such seats are
available.

e. You are allergic and want a special diet prepared
for you on the plane—no salt, flour or milk
products.

5. After each person has purchased his or her ticket,
participants return to the circle where each packs his
or her suitcase (in pantomime). Ask each person to
think of one thing to pack that no one else would
think of—something special, something unusual.

6. Discuss those special, unusual things that were
packed. What do those choices reveal about the
characters?

The Flight

7. With seats arranged airplane fashion, participants
take their seats for the flight to Mexico. Volunteers
should be chosen for the stewardess or steward, cap-
tain and co-captain. The stewardess or steward
might pass out cups of juice and/or cookies for the
in-flight lunch. The leader may want to be the
steward's assistant to facilitate action, or she could
be the group's tour director.

8. If there are several people who enjoy singing or telling jokes, there could be a talent presentation on board to take the place of the in-flight movie because the camera has experienced mechanical difficulties.

9. Before disembarking, the leader may want to get travelers' opinions about the airline:

   a. How do you feel about the airline?
   b. Do they really try to please the customer?

The Bullfight

10. When the plane lands, mariachi music could begin. The leader asks the group to imagine that they have checked into the hotel, unpacked their luggage and are setting off to a bullfight. Ask for a volunteer for the bullfighter. Give the bullfighter a cape. Improvise a bullfight scene. Will the bull win? Will the fighter win? Will the bull chase the fighter out of the ring? Will the fighter and the bull become friends? Perhaps after the first pair have done their bit, another pair would like to volunteer. Meantime, the crowd can be commenting on the bullfight, shouting "ole" and tossing "rose petals" into the ring.

The Market

11. The leader explains that the room has been changed into a marketplace and that for a moment, he or she wants each participant to imagine that he or she is a merchant trying to sell something. Discuss what might be sold, e.g., bananas, chickens, sombreros, flowers. Ask each participant to ready his or her stall (in pantomime). Invite them to work on hawking their wares.

12. Ask for volunteers to be the shoppers. Then improvise a scene in which the vendors are trying to attract the attention of the shoppers, in which shoppers and vendors bargain, etc. Later, shoppers might want to become vendors and other vendors might wish to become shoppers.

13. Introduce conflict by announcing that all your American Express checks are missing. What will you do? Discuss various courses of action. You might play out scenes in which the group visits the police, the American Express office. They might decide to capture the bandit themselves or perhaps the checks will be found.

Conclusion:

1. Discuss what it is about travel that makes it so exciting and appealing to people.

2. Why does the spirit of wanderlust persist?

3. This drama might culminate in actually planning and making a short trip (to the zoo, a museum, a play) together from the home or senior center.

4. What influences do we see on life in the United States from our neighbor to the south, Mexico?

Chapter 7

SESSION PLANS

Following are a number of sample session plans. They are quite detailed to further demonstrate how the techniques discussed in Chapter 6 can be implemented.

The format of each plan is as follows:

1. *Objectives*: These indicate the kinds of behavior hoped for from the participants during the session. Such objectives are helpful to the leader in evaluating the success of the session.
2. *Before the session*: Materials and equipment to be located before the session begins. Room arrangements to be made.
3. *Introduction*: During the first five to ten minutes the session theme is introduced and interest is aroused through the leader's questions and use of music, pictures, objects, etc. Games and ice breakers may also be used.
4. *Development*: The major portion of the session in which players become involved in activities related to the theme such as pantomime, role playing, improvisation or story dramatization. Questions and discussions are interwoven throughout.
5. *Conclusion*: The last five to ten minutes of the session in which participants are guided to discuss their thoughts and feelings about the drama. This is a time to probe for depth and meaning and to reflect on the joy of creating together.

Plans are arranged roughly in order of difficulty with the easiest appearing first. They include:

1. The Auction	6. The Restaurant
2. Marigolds	7. The Beach Party
3. Market Research	8. The Lighthouse
4. Cookies	9. The Quilt
5. Department Store	

Photo by Dawn Murray

THE AUCTION

Objectives:
1. Verbalize comfortably in a simple role playing situation.

2. Create an imaginary history for a real object.

3. Create dialogue for the auctioneer.

4. Play the role of a customer at an auction, bidding on various items.

Before the Session:
1. Assemble various items to be auctioned off. Give priority to items that are interesting looking, humorous or unusual, e.g., Mrs. Butterworth's bottle, sun umbrella, riding stick, music box, elaborate hat, humorous bank, cactus plant. (Note: Since these items will be claimed and carried away by participants, you may wish to ask staff members for white elephants.)

2. Purchase play money or xerox play money so that each participant can receive several thousand "dollars."

3. Make a large construction paper or tagboard sign that reads, "AUCTION TODAY."

4. Locate a boater or other interesting hat for leader to wear (optional).

5. Make enough lemonade for all. Have paper cups ready.

Introduction:
1. Have chairs assembled audience fashion, with an aisle down the middle. As participants arrive, escort them to their seats, making a personal comment to each and welcoming each to the auction.

2. After everyone has arrived, explain that all of the amazing items at the front of the crowd are going to be auctioned off and that you are just waiting for the auctioneer. (Each time you say you are waiting

for the auctioneer, glance somewhat nervously at your watch and then around the room as if you can't imagine where he or she might be. The leader is using a bit of role playing here.)

Development:

1. Invite participants to take a good look at the items being auctioned and to start thinking about what items they might want to buy.

2. Distribute "money" to each participant explaining that they may use it to bid at the auction.

3. After glancing about for the auctioneer a few more times, explain that it looks like the auctioneer isn't going to show up. Suggest that to avoid wasting time, you will auction off the items if participants will help you think of things to say about each item.

4. Take an item, for example a pirate head cookie jar, and elicit a description from the audience. Possible questions the leader might ask are:

   a. Who do you think originally owned this cookie jar?

   b. If you had the cookie jar, what unusual uses could you put it to?

   c. What do you think it is made of?

5. Get ideas on several items to be auctioned.

6. After getting input on how items could be described, begin auction, using as many ideas from the audience as possible. E.g., "I have here an antique cookie jar. It was owned by one of the wealthiest merchants in town and can be used to store all your gold. What am I bid?" If bidding is slow at first, you may ask specific people, "Mrs. Jones, I'm sure you could really use this jar. Will you give me $100.00 for it? O.K. now, I have a bid of $100.00 from Mrs. Jones, who will give me $200.00?"

7. Give items to highest bidder.

Conclusion:

1. Thank everyone for attending the auction and for helping you out of a jam when the auctioneer didn't arrive.

2. Distribute lemonade.

3. While drinking lemonade, speculate about what unusual uses each participant might put their new acquisitions to.

4. Discuss auctions participants have attended.

5. Discuss why auctions are so popular.

6. Make a personal comment to each participant as he or she leaves the group.

Note:

If the leader prefers, someone else—another staff member, a volunteer, the cook—may be brought in to do the auctioning. It is important to have several more items than the number of persons in the group in order that each may bid and buy one or more.

MARIGOLDS

Objectives:

1. Participants will use senses of touch, smell and sight in planting marigolds.

2. Participants will use sensory recall to discuss gardens they remember.

Before the Session:

1. Assemble enough paper cups, yogurt containers or small flower pots for planting small seedlings.

2. Purchase enough marigold plants so that each participant may have one.

3. Purchase a bag of potting soil large enough so that each participant may plant his or her flower.

4. Assemble newspaper or paper towelling to protect working area, scoop or spoon for soil, watering can,

dish pan and liquid soap for washing hands, paper towelling for drying hands.

Introduction: 1. Greet each participant as he or she arrives. Invite them to sit around a table.

2. Talk about some flower you noticed in your home, or on the way to work or in a flower shop. Ask participants what flowers they like best and why.

3. Go into pantomime. "Imagine you're in a flower garden":

   a. Smell the roses in front of you.

   b. Now lean down and smell those dandelions. Pick one. Rub it under your chin to see if you like butter, the way we did when we were kids.

   c. How about planting some flower seeds? First dig a little hole in the ground. Now put the seeds in. Cover them over with dirt. Don't forget to water them.

4. Distribute planting materials and assist each participant in planting his or her own marigold. While participants are planting, side coach to heighten sensory awareness. You might draw attention to the feel and color of the soil, length and strength of the roots, color and smell of the flowers, the way the soil soaks up the water, etc. Perhaps read flower poems while participants are planting their marigolds.

5. Talk about what the marigolds look like, what they smell like, what they feel like.

6. Recall gardens participants have worked in or seen on trips, e.g., famous gardens (Versailles) or herb gardens.

7. Other possible topics for discussion:

   a. Trials and problems of gardening

   b. Rewards of a garden

c. Disappointments with gardens or gardening

d. Favorite flowers—why?

Conclusion: 1. Discuss why people all over the world seem to love flowers. Why are flowers so often used for special occasions?

2. Invite participants to take their marigolds with them and to care for them.

3. Make a personal comment to each participant as he or she leaves the session.

MARKET RESEARCH

Objectives: 1. Use imagination to create new name for product.

2. Use sense of smell to develop opinion about various scents.

3. Discuss reaction to various scents.

Before the Session:

1. Fill three to four small capped plastic bottles with perfume, one scent to each bottle. Try to choose widely differing scents. It would be especially effective if some had fairly recognizable odors, e.g., lilac, lily of the valley.

2. Locate a brand name perfume for Step 2, Introduction.

3. Have names thought up for all but the test sample, #1–Sweet Rose, #2–Moon Madness, #3–Enchantress. Have small sachets, scented soaps or manufacturer's samples of aftershave and perfume, etc. available to distribute to participants at end of session. (Note: This is not essential but would be a nice finishing touch for the session.)

4. If possible, locate a white smock, lab coat or at least a big apron for the tester to wear in the role of cosmetic scientist.

5. On a 9x12 piece of white paper or tag board, print "BUSY BEE COSMETICS."

Introduction:　　1. As participants arrive, greet each one by name and make a personal comment to each.

2. Explain that you've just bought a new perfume. Spray some on your wrist and ask everyone to sniff it. Ask how they like it. Ask what perfume they like and why. When do they use, have they used perfume? Ask the men what aftershave they like and why.

Development:　　1. Tell participants that the Busy Bee Cosmetics Company (display sign) has asked them to do some market research because the company wants to increase its sales and wants to come out with some new scents.

2. Explain that some of the new scents have already been named, but there is one that has them stumped.

3. Pass around the scents that have been named, one at a time, discussing each after everyone has had a chance to smell it. For example, "Now this perfume, #2, already has a name. I'm going to pass it around and I want each of you to smell it. Think about whether it is a scent you would like to wear. Or if you're a man, think about whether it is a scent you would like your sweetheart to wear."

"Does this perfume remind you of anything? When do you think you might wear it or want your sweetheart to wear it? What kind of person do you think would like to wear this scent?"

"The name the company has given to this is Sweet Rose."

4. Repeat procedure similar to Step 3 with all named scents.

5. Explain that you have now come to the scent that Busy Bee Cosmetics can't name. "This will be a very important test. The company just can't seem to come up with a name for this perfume and we can be very helpful to them."

6. Pass scent around asking everyone to smell it carefully. Discuss with questions similar to those used in Step 3. Discuss name that should be given to the product. Why? Leader may tape record or take notes on session so information can be "sent" to Busy Bee Cosmetics Company. (Note: An aftershave lotion rather than a perfume could be used for the naming phase if there are men in the group.)

Conclusion: 1. Talk about which scent participants liked best and why.

2. Comment that it is interesting that everyone, even Busy Bee Cosmetics and Johnson's Wax, needs advice and help from others sometimes. Discuss why companies spend time and money to get opinions from people before introducing a new product.

3. Let each participant put a dab of the perfume of their choice on.

4. Distribute small token from "the company."

5. Make a personal comment to each participant as he or she leaves.

COOKIES

Objectives: 1. Share memories associated with baking and the smells of baking.

2. Improvise a scene with a partner after the who, what, when, where, why are given.

3. Describe imagined sensory experiences.

Before the Session:
1. Find an old fashioned cookie can.

2. Assemble pictures of cookies or utensils for making cookies if desired.

3. Bake or purchase a batch of cookies to share at the conclusion of the session.

Introduction: 1. Hold up the cookie jar and ask participants what kind of cookies they would put in it to fill it up.

2. Ask if anyone's mother had a special jar or can where she kept cookies. What did it look like? Where did she keep it?

3. Discuss what the kitchen smelled like when cookies were being baked.

4. Ask if anyone can remember helping mother or grandmother or aunt when she was baking or cooking. What kinds of things were done to help?

Development: 1. Make a transition to drama. You might say, "Let's suppose you were a boy or girl who is supposed to bring cookies that you have baked for the school's bake sale. BUT you have never made a cookie before. So you go to your grandmother who is a super good cook and ask her to teach you. Maybe she will even share her secret recipe with you. You are in kind of a hurry because you have to do your homework and bake the cookies tonight, so it may be a bit difficult to pay attention.

2. Assign partners, one to be the child, one to be the grandmother. (Partners should be sitting next to each other and with some distance between them and other pairs.)

3. Set the scene: "Grandmother, imagine you are in your kitchen. Everything is in reach—the stove, cupboards, refrigerator, the table just in front of you. When I knock three times, that means your young friend is at the door and the scene is ready to start. We'll all talk at once so don't worry about anyone but just the two of you. Any questions?"

4. Complicate the situation. Tell each of the grandmothers, secretly, that they are to use non-standard measures, e.g., a pinch of this, a handful of that.

5. All pairs play their scenes simultaneously. Later, you may wish to allow each pair to share a part of their scene with the group.

6. Discuss the scene just played:

To child learners—

a. Do you think you will have any problems in making cookies like grandmother made them. How so?

b. Did she let you help in any way?

c. How did being in a hurry make it difficult to listen?

To grandmother teachers—

a. Did you have any problems in keeping the child's attention? How did you handle this?

b. What problems do you think the child will have in making cookies by him or herself?

7. Make a transition to Scene Two. You might say, "Now let's suppose it's a day later and the children have made their cookies for the bake sale. Of course all the grandmothers are coming to the sale. One

rule of the sale is that each seller must provide a small sample of their cookies to help people decide which to buy.

"Grandmothers, you can buy from anyone except the child you taught. What will you consider before you buy any cookies?

What is the school going to do with the money they make on the sale? How will you hawk your wares? (Their chants can include price, ingredients, color, size, aroma, shape, decoration, etc. For example, "Sugar cookies here, only five cents. Any shape you want. Come and taste." Or, "If you like dates, you'll love these date bars. Chewy and gooey, just right for a late evening snack.")

Ask sellers to sit or stand beside a chair to represent their sales booth. Buyers can move from booth to booth.

"When I give the signal (flick of lights, the word 'begin,' or hand signal, etc.), all sellers start to call out to the crowd something special about your cookies."

8. The group enacts Scene Two.

Conclusion: 1. Discuss the scene:

   a. Buyers, what did you notice about samples? What tastes were especially good?

   b. Sellers, how did you feel about the customers? Did they seem to appreciate the samples? What did they say?

   c. Buyers, what did you notice about the way the sellers displayed their cookies? What did they do to make it attractive?

   d. Did you feel the prices were fair? Reasonable? Too high?

e. Did you feel the sellers were pleasant? Patient? Helpful?

f. In what way were the buyers different from one another?

g. In what way were the sellers different from one another?

2. Discuss what it is about school bake sales and socials that makes them so popular. What events at the community center or nursing home generate some of the same feelings? Are there other events that might create a feeling of community?

3. Enjoy eating the cookies.

DEPARTMENT STORE

Objectives: 1. Take the role of a character different from oneself.

2. Pantomime using various items in a department store.

3. Verbalize ideas for "selling" various items in the store.

4. Engage in spontaneous dialogue in an improvised scene.

Before the Session:

1. Assemble a collection of "department store items" like outlandish hats, costume jewelry, white elephants.

2. Make a sign reading "Whitehouse Department Store" (or the name of your facility/center).

Introduction: 1. Greet each participant and make a personal comment to each as they arrive.

2. To get things started, ask a progression of questions, such as: "Have you ever worked in a department

store? Do you know anyone who has worked in a department store? Have any funny things ever happened to you in a department store? What is your favorite department to shop in? Why?"

Development: 1. Announce that today everyone in the group is going to have an opportunity to work in a department store, the Whitehouse Department Store. But in order to give all the new employees (the participants) an opportunity to find out what work they like best, they will be trained in various areas first.

2. *Gift Wrapping*
Begin the training in the gift wrapping department where new employees will wrap gifts of various sizes and description (in pantomime). Ask participants to suggest gifts to wrap, e.g., a tiny ring, a mink coat, a tricycle, a crystal bud vase, a wind-up toy that keeps wandering off. Have everyone wrap the same item simultaneously to facilitate side coaching. "Is your ring a diamond? Emerald? What color is the box? What kind of paper will you choose?" etc.

3. *Sales Training*
Move on to the retail sales training. Working in pairs, one participant in each pair will be the salesperson and the other will be the picky, hard to please customer. Give each pair one item. The salesperson will try to satisfy the customer while the customer does his or her best to find fault. After a time, suggest that participants change roles. If participants have been together for awhile and feel comfortable in the drama group, spotlighting (see p. 26) could be used.

4. *Floor Demonstration*
The next phase of the training is being a floor demonstrator. Instruct each participant to decide on an imaginary product to demonstrate, e.g., an automatic potato peeler, dog washing machine, electric peanut butter spreader. Ask for a few examples from

the group and discuss the special features and operating instructions for the product. At a given signal, all participants will begin simultaneously demonstrating their products using pantomime and improvising their sales pitch. (See p. 40.) Following the simultaneous demonstrations, spotlighting could be used.

5. *Customer Relations*

The final phase of training is customer relations. Participants again work in pairs, with one person in each pair being the customer relations person while the other is an irate customer attempting to return an item. Before the pair work begins, discuss store policy and protocol on returning items: check condition of mechandise, need for sales slip to accompany returned merchandise, assess validity of reasons for return. After a time, allow participants to switch roles.

Conclusion:

1. Ask participants which job they found easiest and why. Which was the hardest?

2. Discuss whether the experience made anyone feel any differently about salespeople.

3. Discuss which job each participant would like to do and why.

4. How are department stores today different from those when you were growing up?

THE RESTAURANT

Objectives: 1. Play the role of customers or employees of a restaurant.

2. Create dialogue for man on the street interview.

3. Pantomime various activities in restaurant.

4. Participate verbally in planning restaurant scenario.

Before the Session:

1. Prepare menus (a sample menu with 3-4 choices is best).

    Example:

    ITALIAN VILLAGE
    Spaghetti
    Lasagne
    Veal Parmesan

2. Assemble "costumes" such as hats for customers, boutonnieres for men, apron for waitress. A flower for each woman to pin on would be nice, too.

3. Arrange a circle of chairs for the beginning of the session (one chair ready for each participant).

4. Set up table (or tables) with brightly colored tablecloths (perhaps a red check), flowers, a wine bottle with a candle in it.

5. Prepare an 8½" x 5½" (one-half sheet typing paper) "handbill" advertising the restaurant.

    Example:

    NEW! NEW! NEW!
    ITALIAN VILLAGE

    OPENING SEPTEMBER 15

    SPECIALIZING IN
    LASAGNE * SPAGHETTI
    VEAL PARMESAN

    COME AND SEE US!

6. If there is not a telephone in the room, bring one in (a toy one would do).

7. Other materials: hand mirror
record of Italian music
wine list
Italian cookies

Introduction: 1. Welcome each participant to the session. Be sure to look at each person—eye contact is important. Be sure comments are sincere.

2. Explain that you've received an interesting flyer and want to share it with the group. Pass the flyer around. Discuss the flyer, e.g., "Has anyone been to an Italian restaurant? What was it like? What kind of food did they serve?"

3. Simulate being interrupted by a phone call. After you hang up, say something like, "Oh, wait until I tell you the news. We've been invited to sample the food at the Italian Village. The owner wants to get some testimonials and he needs somebody to try the food out. Isn't that exciting?"

4. Make a list of what personnel would be found at the restaurant, e.g., hat check girl, cashier, maitre'd, waiter or waitress. Ask for volunteers for various positions and indicate places for them to be.

5. Distribute hats and boutonnieres or flowers (to pin on as corsage) to remaining participants. They may want to look in hand mirror.

Development: 1. Pantomime getting ready to go to the restaurant, e.g., brushing teeth, men shaving, women doing nails, fixing hair. Pantomime various tasks of restaurant personnel, e.g., serving, taking orders, clearing tables.

2. Go to restaurant and have maitre'd seat guests. Italian music can now be played.

3. Waitress brings menus and participants discuss choice. (Note: Leader may want to play role of waitress to keep things flowing smoothly.)

4. Waitress takes orders. Pantomime writing them down.

5. If a participant doesn't ask for the wine list, offer the wine list. Discuss choice.

6. Waitress serves food.

7. Pantomime eating food. Dinner table chatter.

8. Suggest dancing. Perhaps someone will want to provide entertainment.

9. Leader says, "Imagine now that I'm a newspaper reporter and that I've come to get your opinion about this restaurant." Interview participants asking questions about prices, service, quality of food, pasta, wine, sauces, meats, salads, etc.

Conclusions:

1. Talk about what each person enjoyed most. Discuss what makes a restaurant pleasant to go to and what would make you decide not to return.

2. Collect hats. Comment on some nice piece of participation as each person returns his or her hat.

3. Say goodbye to each person and invite them to come again.

THE BEACH PARTY

Objectives: 1. Pantomime eating, putting on lotion, swimming and other beach-related activities.

2. Role play members of picnic groups at beach.

3. Participate with group in warm-up games and discussion.

4. Invent reasons why two groups might want the same site.

5. Use problem solving skills in discussing resolution of the beach scene conflict.

Before the Session:

1. Try to get a recording of "By the Sea" or "In the Good Old Summertime" to play as participants arrive.

2. Find a colorful plastic beach ball for "Information Please."

Introduction: 1. Greet each participant as he or she arrives.

2. Play "Information Please" (p. 14). Some questions that might be asked are, "In the summertime, I like to _____," "The best thing about warm weather is _____," "When I go to the beach, I like to _____."

3. Leader says something like, "Gee, all that talk about summer and picnics and the beach makes me feel like taking a break. Wouldn't it be fun if we could just take off right now and have a picnic on the beach? Let's see. What are some of the foods we could bring?"

4. As participants name foods, leader amplifies the contribution and invites everyone to remember how watermelon, for example, tastes, feels and smells. "Remember how juicy watermelon can be. I remember eating it and having the juice just running down my arms. And spitting the seeds! That's the most

fun. Let's try it. Here, I'll slice a piece for each of you." Leader slices imaginary watermelon and gives a slice to each participant along with an imaginary napkin. "O.K., everybody. Take a big bite. Watch out for seeds."

5. Remember other foods that might be taken on a beach picnic and pantomime preparing, eating, smelling or touching them.

Development: 1. "All that talk about food has made me wish we really were having a picnic at the beach. Listen, let's imagine that this room is the beach and that we're all here having a good time."

2. Pantomime opening tubes or bottles of suntan lotion and rubbing it on shoulders, arms, etc.

3. Pantomime swimming, putting up umbrellas, spreading blankets, tug-of-war or other activities.

4. Invite everyone to gather around the "campfire" to sing songs like "You Are My Sunshine," "Down By the Old Mill Stream," etc. If you have access to someone who plays the guitar, this would be a welcome addition.

5. Pantomime roasting marshmallows.

6. Leader raises questions of what would happen if just as they were really feeling comfortable and relaxed with each other, another group came up and insisted that this spot was reserved for them? Answers might range from, "We'd tell them they'd just have to find another place," to "I'd tell 'em to go jump in the lake," to "We could invite them to join us."

7. After discussing various possibilities, leader might suggest that they play out one of the scenarios, e.g., the first group says they won't move while the second insists that the first group has to move.

8. The leader asks for volunteers to play the roles of those in the new group and guides each group to

decide on their reason for being together at the beach, e.g., family reunion, company picnic, birthday party.

9. If there is an assistant leader or co-leader, he or she can serve as a "spokesperson" for one group while the leader can serve in that capacity for the other, helping to keep dialogue going and promote more interaction.

10. If there is no assistant or co-leader, the leader can keep action going and heighten the tension through questions, e.g., "Why are you interrupting our party?" or "What makes you think this spot is yours?" or "What did you want to use this spot for?"

11. After improvisation has gone on for some time, leader can stop action and ask participants how conflict can be resolved. "What might bring the two groups together? Some kind of external threat? Something that might lure or entice them to join forces? Some emergency that required their help?

12. Group decides which possibilities to play out. Improvisation continues.

Conclusion:

1. Leader guides discussion about what caused the beach scene to end on such a happy note (compromise, willingness to work together).

2. Leader asks how participants felt when they were both arguing over the same area of the beach. How they felt when they agreed to join forces.

3. Discuss what they enjoyed most about today's session.

4. Sing a group song.

5. Make a personal comment to each participant as he or she leaves.

THE LIGHTHOUSE

Objectives: 1. Pantomime various beach activities, alone and in pairs.

2. Verbally recall previous "beach" experiences.

3. Create a community environment through imagined details.

4. Plan scenes involving interaction between towns-people and lighthouse keeper.

5. Improvise scenes involving conflict between towns-people and lighthouse keeper.

Before the Session:

1. If possible, find a record with seashore sounds or some mood music like Debussy's *La Mer*.

2. Prepare a "letter" from the government to inform the lighthouse keeper that the lighthouse is to be closed and that he or she will have to move. The sample letter might look like this:

Dear Lighthouse Keeper:

This letter is to inform that you will soon be relieved of your duties. This lighthouse will be con-verted to automatic mechanical management. We will no longer need someone living at the lighthouse 24 hours a day. We request that you vacate the premises within 30 days of receipt of this letter.

Sincerely,

Director of Lighthouse Services
United States Coast Guard

3. If possible, prepare a small box filled with sand.

Introduction: 1. Greet each participant as he or she arrives. Make a personal comment to each or ask a question of each.

2. The leader passes the box of sand around, inviting the participants to put their fingers in it and to let

the sand sift through their fingers to recall the beach environment.

3. With the participants seated in a circle, leader asks them to share their experiences at the beach—perhaps at the ocean, perhaps at a lake.

Development:

1. While music is playing, the leader guides the participants through a variety of beach-related pantomimes:

   a. Digging with their hands in the sand

   b. Letting the sand sift through their fingers

   c. Building a sand castle

   d. Looking for and collecting shells

   e. Unpacking a picnic lunch (later, participants may discuss what was in their particular lunch)

   f. Playing beach ball, frisbee or other games on the beach (participants may work in partners and add improvised dialogue)

2. Leader asks participants to imagine they are employees of a warehouse that supplies an isolated lighthouse keeper with fresh supplies every two or three months. The leader takes on the role of the new warehouse supervisor and asks the warehouse employees to remember what supplies they took to the lighthouse keeper last trip out. These questions are to challenge them to think very specifically.

   a. "What dried food did we take him the last time?" (beans, prunes, peas, oatmeal, flour.)

   b. "Didn't he ask us to bring some seasonings and flavorings? Do you recall what they were? (Catsup, mustard, vanilla, onions.)

   c. "What clothing did he say he needed?" (Long Johns, slicker, boots.)

    d. I remember he said he wanted something more to read. What books or magazines shall we bring him? (*Field & Stream, Life, Reader's Digest.*)

    e. He has a lot of time on his hands. Any other ideas for his leisure time? (Crossword puzzles, stationery, wood for whittling, a bird to keep him company.)

    f. Do you suppose he needs some batteries for the radio? Kerosene for the lantern? Fishhooks? Boat oars?

3. After indicating where the boats are, the leader, in role, directs the workers to load supplies onto the boats asking each to indicate what they have brought.

4. Before setting off for the lighthouse, the leader may ask for local news to share with the lighthouse keeper. The leader might say something like, "One of the things your former boss told me was how much Mr. Johnson liked news about what's going on in the village. Does anybody have a tidbit of news to bring him?" The leader could get the ball rolling by suggesting such tidbits as:

—Mrs. Roth had twin boys.
—The school superintendent ran off with the public health nurse.
—Old Nate Stevens is still raising a ruckus every Friday evening.
—The City Hall is finally getting a new coat of paint.

5. Leaders ask participants to imagine that they are getting into their boats to deliver the supplies to the lighthouse. Pantomime rowing a boat.

6. Leader produces "letter" which tells lighthouse keeper he or she will have to move. Discuss how the lighthouse keeper might feel about such a move, why the government might be closing the light-

house, and what might help the keeper feel better about having to move.

7. Ask for a volunteer to take the role of the light-house keeper. Plan and play improvised scenes such as the following:

   a. The group arrives, bringing supplies. After every-thing has been unloaded, someone presents the lighthouse keeper with the letter.

   b. The lighthouse keeper refuses to go and tells the group about what the lighthouse has meant to him or her.

   c. The group tries to convince the lighthouse keeper that it is really best for him or her to leave.

   d. The scene is resolved.

Conclusion: 1. With the participants seated in a circle, discuss what things each enjoyed most about today's session.

2. Discuss why it was difficult for the lighthouse keeper to leave the lighthouse. Discuss how participants think the lighthouse keeper will feel after moving and how members of the community could help.

3. Relate dilemma of lighthouse keeper to the personal experience of the senior participants. For example, having to move against your will, leaving the home you have lived in for many years, having govern-ment agencies make your decisions.

4. Make a personal comment to each of the participants as they leave.

THE QUILT

Objectives: 1. To recall early experiences.

2. To use imagination in creating dramatic situations.

3. To identify with the feelings of a character in a scene.

4. To develop spontaneity in verbal expression.

5. To enjoy the give and take of interaction with others.

Before the Session:

Locate a patchwork quilt, preferably one that is old and worn. A crazy quilt is recommended, for these often have names and dates embroidered in the patches which give an authenticity to the quilt.

Introduction: 1. Greet each participant and make a personal comment to each as he or she arrives.

2. Start the session with a series of questions:

    a. Do you remember having spelling bees when you were in school? Did you enjoy them? Can you remember the hardest word you ever had to spell? What rules did you have to follow? Do you think people learned to spell better back then than today?

    b. Were there any other bees that people participated in?

    c. What were these like? What were the purposes? (husking bees, quilting bees)

Development: 1. Show the quilt. Invite group to gather around so that they can see and touch. Tell them that the life of the quilt is a mystery which can be unlocked through the use of their imagination. Draw out ideas with the following questions:

    a. What can you tell about the quilt by feeling it? Smelling it?

    b. What do your eyes tell you about the quilt?

    c. When do you think this quilt may have been made?

    d. Do you suppose it was made for some particular occasion? By what kind of person?

    e. What were some of the happiest moments in the life of the quilt?

    f. What was its narrowest escape?

    g. Who do you think loved it the most?

    h. Was there anyone who wanted to get rid of it?

    i. What was the quilt's greatest disappointment?

    j. What was its best kept secret?

    k. What was the major turning point in its life?

Planning the Scenes:

1. List the events that the group wishes to include in the drama of the quilt's life.

    a. Arrange the events in chronological order.

    b. Ask participants if they prefer to start with the most recent event and move backwards in time or if they would rather begin at the time the quilt was made.

2. Structure the content for the first scene to be played. The leader may select certain ideas and guide the group to make other decisions. Decisions to be made include:

    a. Where does the scene take place?

    b. Who are the characters? What are their goals? How are they related?

    c. What happens? What is the problem? Are there obstacles?

Casting and Playing:

1. Choose cast from volunteers. Try planning a very short scene several times, each time with a different cast, before attempting longer scenes. It is often helpful if the leader takes a minor role so she can promote interaction and support the belief of others in the scene. But the group should not become dependent on the leader to carry the scene.

2. *Discussing the scene*
   This portion of the session can develop observational and critical skills of both the players and the audience. The discussion should be focused on positive and constructive remarks and deal with the characters involved, not with the personality of the real players. Questions to players might include:

   a. (to players) What did your character want in this scene?

   b. (to players) Did anything or anyone stand in the way of your achieving what you wanted? How did this affect the outcome of the scene? How did your character feel about this?

   Questions to the whole group might include:

   a. How did these people feel about one another?

   b. How did they relate to the quilt? Was it valued? Why?

   c. What moments were most real, most believable to you?

   d. What suggestions do you have for changing or improving the scene before we choose a new cast and play it again?

3. *Replaying the scene*
   Choose another cast and replay.

Conclusion: In addition to evaluating the last playing of the scene, this is a time to relate the drama to the players' lives in some larger way. Questions might include:

a. Do you have an heirloom that is important to you or your family? Have any heirlooms been lost or destroyed?

b. Why is it that things which belonged to our parents or grandparents become so precious to us?

c. Shall we go on next time to play out more events in the life of the quilt, or do you want to start a new topic?

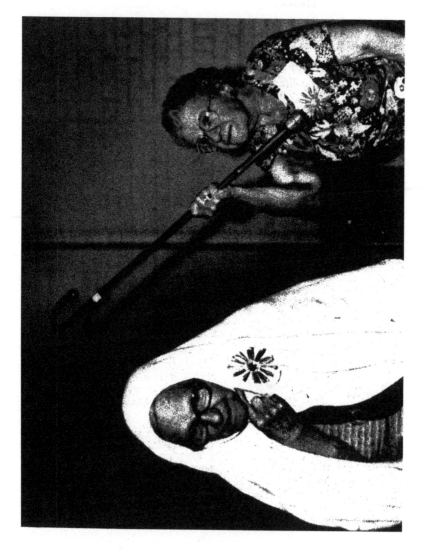

Chapter 8

LITERATURE FOR DRAMATIZATION

Literature can provide a rich source of material for drama. Through someone else's story we can take on another role and face fears, conflicts or problems that may be similar in nature to ours and yet less threatening because they have been removed from our lives.

The Good Samaritan, for example, deals with a pedestrian being attacked by muggers—a very real problem for today's elderly. But some of the angst is removed from the situation because the story is set in Biblical times in a country far away. When the story is translated into the dramatic mode, players can begin to work out frustrations and fears by taking the roles of the traveler and the thugs.

Selecting Literature

Stories can be chosen which relate to the time of childhood or to other real-life experiences. Stories can carry you to places you've never been before. Stories can fulfill wishes for the romantic, the far away, the bizarre. Stories can touch off memory, spark conversation, lead into drama.

Through the metaphor of the role, situations which are too real, too traumatic in everyday life can be faced. Players can project their feelings onto their role in someone else's story. They can reprocess their feelings through the drama. Because literature, and consequently the drama based on it, can project forward and backward, participants can relive their past and anticipate the future. They can dispel the pain of the former and their anxiety about the latter.

In addition, the use of stories as the basis for the drama session can provide security for the drama leader. Stories provide a dependable structure with a beginning, middle and end. Characters are delineated and related to each other through the story line. Settings are described, action is narrated and dialogue is included. Not all stories, however, are suitable for dramatization and several factors should be taken into consideration.

Length

Choose very short stories at first, preferably those with only one scene. This allows the whole story to be read, discussed and played out in one session. Examples of good short, short stories are Aesop's Fables, "A Pound of Kasha" from *Stories for Jewish Juniors*, and "Landladies" from Langston Hughes' *The Best of Simple*.

Longer stories of two or three scenes can be used after the first experience. "The Good Samaritan," "Androcles and the Lion" (from Aesop), "Baucis and Philemon" and "The Man Who Made Trees Blossom" from Philip Payne's *Legends and Drama*, and O. Henry's "The Cop and the Anthem" would work well for beginners. In reading or telling the story, you may want to omit portions that detract from the action to be dramatized including excessive descriptions of characters or settings. Sub-plots may also be deleted, at least in the playing.

Subject Matter and Theme

Above all, the subject matter should be of interest to the seniors and the leader. Whether the topic be humorous or serious, historical or current, realistic or fanciful, it must have the potential to sustain the involvement of the group. If the leader does not enjoy the story, the group is not likely to enjoy it either.

The literature chosen should be worthwhile. It should be well crafted and have universal meaning. The central idea or theme should be one that merits consideration and stimulates discussion.

The story of "The Secret Life of Walter Mitty," for example, deals with something close to the hearts of all of us—coping with the desire to be someone or somewhere we are not through daydreams. This is particularly true if we find ourselves "locked" into situations that irritate us or give us pain. The juxtaposition of fantasy and reality in the story gives us a model. We can play the daydreams just as they appear in the story or we can make up other daydreams. The group can re-enact Mitty's fantasy as the brilliant submarine commander or they might be inspired by his daydreams to share and dramatize their own. Literature becomes a model for our discussion and enactment. We are true to the author's meaning, we replicate the genre, but we open out the story to include our own lives.

Dramatic Action

Stories tell about life; drama shows life. In the novel or short story, the author can tell us through narrative what the characters are feeling or thinking. In a drama, we learn about the feelings and thoughts of characters from what they say and do.

Since drama shows instead of tells, the leader must be careful to choose a story that has strong dramatic action. Generally speaking, dramatic action results when one or more characters with a strong goal or intention struggle against other characters or forces for success.

Just as people in real life have goals, so should characters in a scene or play. Each character behaves in a certain way because he or she wants something. When the needs of two or more people are in opposition or when obstacles stand in the way of a character realizing his or her goal, conflict results. The conflict gives rise to dramatic action. Without conflict, the scene is flat, dull and uninteresting.

Conflict may be found within an individual character, between characters or between the characters and outside physical forces. However the conflict is manifested, though, it is through identification with a character's struggle to overcome obstacles to reach his or her goal that the player experiences the emotional release that makes drama so satisfying.

Joan of Arc, for example, wants to drive the English from French soil. Although she has God, the Dauphin and the French army on her side, there are equally strong forces set against her. The British army, of course, has no intention of leaving. And the Catholic church is outraged that she claims to have heard directly from God. The conflict is gripping and inescapable. A dramatization based on this kind of story is bound to work.

Characters and Dialogue

In general choose stories with interesting characters. Most short stories will provide some background information about the characters such as age; physical condition; occupation; family, social or religious background; attitudes and relationships. But don't rule out fables or parables as the basis for drama just because they provide very little background information. The insights and vast life experience of the senior adult can be brought into play to round out one-dimensional characters.

It is a good idea to choose a story that has several characters so that everyone in the drama group can participate. On the other hand, characters can always be added. In the Good Samaritan, the number of robbers in the band of thieves can easily grow. A scene could be added to introduce the victim's wife and children. Many different travelers can pass by before the Good Samaritan shows up. Characters and scenes can be added so long as the basic integrity of the story is preserved.

As the players consider the characters, as they compare them to people they have known in their own lives, as they begin to bring them to life, they not only find themselves in the characters but they bring new meaning to their understanding of what it is to be human. As they discover ways in which they are like or unlike the characters they play, as they consider whether a character changes during the course of a story, as they decide how to translate the story from the literary to the dramatic mode, they increase their powers of perception.

While the story upon which a dramatization is based may contain much well written dialogue, the leader should discourage any attempts at memorization or strict adherence to the actual text. If the story presents vivid characters with strong identifiable goals, and if the action grows naturally out of these goals, the players will be able to create their own dialogue spontaneously. Each time a scene is played, it will be fresh and different.

Literature for Drama: A Checklist

If you can answer yes to the following questions, you know you have chosen literary materials that can lead to satisfying improvised drama.

Subject Matter

1. Will the subject matter of the literature interest and sustain involvement of seniors?
2. Are you, as leader, enthusiastic about the possibilities of the material?
3. Does the subject relate in some way to the seniors' life experience and/or will the subject move them into a new area of experience?
4. Is the subject treated in a way that is acceptable to the group?

Theme

1. Does the central idea or theme merit consideration of the group?
2. Does it touch on some universal aspect of life?
3. Does it relate directly or indirectly to a current concern of seniors?

Length of Material

1. Can the material be translated into drama in a reasonable number of sessions?
2. Can cuts be made in the number of incidents without destroying the story line? If desired, can the subplot be excised without damaging the main story line?
3. Can lengthy descriptions of character or setting be eliminated?
4. Can the story be read or told to the group in sections?

Dramatic Action and Structure

1. Does the material have an identifiable beginning, middle and end?
2. Do the main characters have strong goals?
3. Do the main characters face obstacles (human or otherwise) as they strive to attain their goals?
4. Is the conflict of the story resolved in a believable way?
5. Is the action of the story carried out primarily in overt, physical terms? Can important inner/covert action be eliminated or translated to overt action?
6. Does the action seem well motivated?
7. Can the action be carried out by your particular group of seniors?

Character

1. Are there clearly defined characters? If there are too many characters so that none stand out clearly, can some be eliminted?
2. Are there enough characters to keep the interest of your group? If not, can other characters be meaningfully added?
3. Do you learn about characters mostly from what they do? Are they also revealed by what they say and what others say?
4. Are character relationships clear? Are there differences among characters?

5. Do characters seem true to life? Are they believable?
6. Are the goals of the characters clear? Strong? Do you understand why they do what they do?
7. Will your group of seniors be able to identify with and enjoy playing these characters? Will they find the characters challenging to play? Will they find enough depth in the characters?

Dialogue

1. Does the dialogue grow out of the action? Further the action?
2. Does the dialogue sound like it fits the characters? Does it reflect the characters' background?
3. If there is little or no dialogue, is the action of the story strong enough to help the group create spontaneous dialogue?
4. Will it be necessary to add a narrator to interpret the inner thoughts and feelings of the characters?

Before You Present the Story

Before you present the story to your group, read it several times. Decide upon any cuts and changes needed. Read the story several times out loud, visualizing the setting, the characters and the action. Become thoroughly familiar with it. Determine what parts of the story you will read and what parts you will tell in your own words. Decide how you will introduce the story. Will you use an object, an action, a picture, music? What questions will you use?

Outline the basic sequence of events of the story so that the story line is simplified and clear to you. A simple plot analysis, like a road map, can show you where the story is going. The elements are like a skeleton, the bare bones on which to elaborate. Analysis of the structure will point up the strengths and weaknesses of the literature in terms of its suitability for transformation into drama. Not all narrative fiction, poetry or other forms of literature have a dramatic structure, but with elaboration and extension, they can still form the basis of dramatization.

Identifying Dramatic Structure

First of all, identify the aspects of dramatic structure that are present in the literature. The beginning consists of background information (*exposition*) and the action that sets the story in motion (*precipitating ac-*

tion). The exposition usually establishes when and where the story takes place. Major characters are introduced. Any action prior to the beginning of the story is described. The precipitating action gets the play going. The main character(s) have a problem or are plunged into trouble which starts the main conflict of the story.

The middle consists of several *complications* and the *crisis*. The complications are a series of events in which the main characters attempt to achieve their goal against opposing forces. The crisis is the turning point, the last most crucial complication when the main characters must win or lose.

The end consists of the *resolution* in which the conflict is resolved, and the *conclusion* is a return to the state of equilibrium in which all loose ends are knit together.

If we analyze "The Good Samaritan" for dramatic structure, our efforts might look like Figure 1.

Identifying Dramatic Elements

Another way to look at the story is to identify the dramatic elements, particularly the setting (where), characters (who), and action (what). This will assist the leader in breaking the story down into playable scenes. This step also helps to clarify what information is and is not provided by the story and shows where elaboration will be needed. In Figure 2 we see that "The Good Samaritan" has three scenes, but only two settings. The thieves appear in only one scene, the Samaritan in two and the traveler in three.

Developing and Elaborating the Story

In preparing to dramatize a short story, particularly a parable like "The Good Samaritan," it is necessary to flesh out the characters, their motivation and relationships, to visualize the details of the setting and to elaborate the dramatic action. The leader's careful phrasing of questions will signal that there is no right or wrong answer and should promote a number of responses. Questions should encourage participants to relate their past experiences, the books they've read and the films they've seen to the characters in "The Good Samaritan." Other questions should press them to use their imagination in making inferences about the behavior and motivation of the Levite and the thieves. As details of the

Figure 1

STORY - "THE GOOD SAMARITAN"

And, behold, a certain lawyer stood up, and tempted him, saying, Master, what shall I do to inherit eternal life?

He said unto him, What is written in the law? how readest thou?

And he answering said, Thou shalt love the Lord thy God with all thy heart, and with all thy soul, and with all thy strength, and with all thy mind; and thy neighbour as thyself.

And he said unto him, Thou hast answered right: this do, and thou shalt live.

But he, willing to justify himself, said unto Jesus, And who is my neighbour?

And Jesus answering said,

A certain man went down from Jerusalem to Jericho, and fell among thieves, which stripped him of his raiment, and wounded him, and departed, leaving him half dead.

And by chance there came down a certain priest that way: and when he saw him, he passed by on the other side. And likewise a Levite, when he was at the place, came and looked on him, and passed by on the other side. But a certain Samaritan, as he journeyed, came where he was: and when he saw him, he had compassion on him, and went to him, and bound up his wounds, pouring in oil and wine, and set him on his own beast, and brought him to an inn, and took care of him.

And on the morrow when he departed, he took out two pence, and gave them to the host, and said unto him, Take care of him, and whatsoever thou spendest more, when I come again, I will repay thee.

Which now of these three, thinkest thou, was neighbour unto him that fell among thieves?

And he said, He that shewed mercy on him. Then Jesus said unto him, Go and be thou like him.

IDENTIFYING DRAMATIC STRUCTURE

BEGINNING

Exposition: A man travels from Jericho to Jerusalem

Precipitating Action: Thieves attack and leave the man to die

MIDDLE

Complication #1: No help comes from the Priest

Complication #2: No help comes from the Levite

Crisis: Will the man live or die?

END

Resolution: Samaritan aids the man and takes him to inn.

Conclusion: Samaritan pays innkeeper and promises further payment if needed.

The initial and final frames to the story may be told by a narrator, dramatized, or omitted.

Figure 2

STORY - "THE GOOD SAMARITAN"

IDENTIFYING DRAMATIC ELEMENTS:

SETTING, CHARACTER, ACTION BY SCENE

SCENE I

And Jesus answering said, A certain man went down from Jerusalem to Jericho, and fell among thieves, which stripped him of his raiment, and wounded him, and departed, leaving him half dead.

SETTING	CHARACTERS	ACTION SEQUENCE
Road from Jerusalem to Jericho	Traveler 3 Thieves	Traveler comes along the road. Thieves surround traveler, take money, clothes. Attack and leave traveler to die.

SCENE II

And by chance there came down a certain priest that way: and when he saw him, he passed by on the other side. And likewise a Levite, when he was at the place, came and looked on him, and passed by on the other side. But a certain Samaritan, as he journeyed, came where he was: and when he saw him, he had compassion on him, and went to him, and bound up his wounds, pouring in oil and wine, and set him on his own beast, and brought him to an inn, and took care of him.

SETTING	CHARACTERS	ACTION SEQUENCE
Same as 1	Traveler Priest Levite Samaritan	Priest sees, avoids traveler by crossing to opposite side of road. Levite reacts in same way. Samaritan sees traveler, stops, cleanses/binds wounds and helps him upon an ass.

SCENE III

And on the morrow when he departed, he took out two pence, and gave them to the host, and said unto him, Take care of him; and whatsoever thou spendest more, when I come again, I will repay thee.

SETTING	CHARACTERS	ACTION SEQUENCE
Inn	Innkeeper Servants Samaritan	Next morning the Samaritan explains that he must leave. Thanks and pays the innkeeper. Promises to return and pay for any further care for the traveler.

setting on the roadway emerge through discussion, participants can see the dust and feel the noon-day heat.

It is through this process of elaboration and detailing via the leaders' questions that players become more involved and feel confident enough to take on the roles. The outline in Figure 3 demonstrates the kind of questions a leader might use to help a group elaborate on the bare bones of a story, to imagine and particularize aspects of the setting, characters and action. Opposite each suggested question appears the purpose, the rationale, for asking the question.

It is best to attempt only one scene at a time and perhaps only one scene from a story. In the beginning, scenes will be played for the group alone. Later, players may want to share their dramatization with another group. The primary purpose, though, is always the enjoyment of the group and the extra dimension of meaning the drama can bring to the participants' lives. A bibliography of literature with possibilities for dramatization can be found in the appendix.

Figure 3

DEVELOPING AND ELABORATING THE STORY "THE GOOD SAMARITAN"

| LEADER'S QUESTIONS | PURPOSE FOR QUESTIONS |

INTRODUCTION

Introduction/Motivation

A. Discuss: Who were the worst neighbors you ever had? What did they do that made them such bad neighbors?

B. Tell story of "The Good Samaritan".

C. Discuss: Have you heard of similar incidents that have happened in modern times? Has anything like this ever happened to you?

A. Introduce subject of neighbors. Stimulate recall of specific incidents.

C. Make connections between past and present. Provide opportunity to share personal experiences. Test interest in modern day application of theme.

SCENE I

1. How do you see the road from Jerusalem to Jericho? Are there trees? hills? houses?

2. What's the weather like today? hot? cloudy?

3. Let's decide why this man is on his way to Jericho—the story doesn't tell us. What is his occupation? Does he travel this way often? What does he carry with him?

4. Is there some reason why he might stop awhile? Who else might come along the roadway?

1. Visualize the setting, fill in details of landscape.

2. Draw out ideas about weather, climate.

3. Need to find a motivation for the man's travels. Can also settle on his occupation, age, state of health, family, etc.

4. This will give the audience a chance to see him before the thieves attack. He might have a brief conversation with another traveler.

161

Figure 3 (continued)

LEADER'S QUESTIONS

5. What do the robbers look like? How many are there? Who is their leader? Do we see them before the traveler does?

6. What do the robbers want? What do they get?

7. Why do they take his clothes? and beat him so unmercifully? Do they use any weapons?

8. How is the attack made? Is it a surprise? Does the man try to resist in any way? How?

9. How can we show that the robbers meant business by their bodies? voices? use of language?

SCENE II

1. Why do you suppose the Priest did not stop to help the traveler? And the Levite, what might have been his reason? Why did they cross to the other side of the roadway?

2. Since none of the characters are shown to speak in the story, how can we show how they feel and what may be going on in their minds?

3. How old is the priest? the Levite? Where are they going? What is on their minds? How do they look and walk differently from each other?

PURPOSE FOR QUESTIONS

5. Need to see the robbers as real people, not just stereotypes. Need to establish at what time they enter the scene.

6. Need to establish whether the traveler has what they are looking for.

7. Need to explore the motivations of the robbers.

8. If the scene is to be played convincingly, these questions need answers.

9. If the players are non-ambulatory, the fight will have to be primarily vocal and will depend very much on language.

SCENE II

1. Many answers are possible but none are given in the story. Try to draw out as many answers as you can and see how the scene plays differently according to different motivations.

2. In everyday life, our feelings toward each other are revealed by non-verbal behavior more than by verbal. Surprise, fear, guilt, loathing, affection, etc., are all shown by our posture, gesture, facial expression.

3. An effort to individualize the two characters and to help them become real to us.

Figure 3 (continued)

| LEADER'S QUESTIONS | PURPOSE FOR QUESTIONS |

4. What business does the Samaritan have in Jericho or in Jerusalem? Does he travel this road often? Does he always befriend others or is this incident special? What does he carry? Does he remind you of anyone?

5. How many ways might the Samaritan reveal his compassion for the traveler? What might he say to the traveler to comfort him?

6. Do you think the traveler should retain consciousness before he is taken to the inn?

7. Since it would be difficult for the Samaritan to pick up the traveler and since there is no donkey, how should we end the scene?

4. Again an effort to give the Samaritan purpose and individuality. Relating him to a real person or a fictional one can help develop a clearer image of him.

5. Abstract qualities like compassion must be translated into actions. Allowing him to speak to the traveler, even if the man is unconscious, will help to make the character more believable.

6. What is more dramatically engaging, to have the man remain unconscious or to allow him to respond to the Samaritan? There is no right or wrong answer, it can be tried either way.

7. Any number of answers are possible here.

SCENE III

1. Has the Samaritan stayed at this inn before? Are he and the innkeeper well acquainted?

2. Does the traveler see the Samaritan pay the inn-keeper? If so, how does he acknowledge his benefactor? If he is still in his room, too ill to get up, how does he find out what has happened? Does it change the intent of the story for the traveler to acknowledge the help?

3. Does the innkeeper have a wife? or children? What would their presence contribute to the scene?

1. Either answer is valid, but the scene will be affected by the decision.

2. It is essential to decide whether or not the traveler appears in this scene. Is his recovery to take months? Are we to learn of his recovery or assume it?

Figure 3 (continued)

LEADER'S QUESTIONS

4. Since the scene is so brief, what might be gained by starting the scene early in the morning with the arrival of a couple of servants in the inn. They might have heard some gossip about a traveler who was dying at the inn.

PURPOSE FOR QUESTIONS

4. Here the leader suggests a way to elaborate on the domestic relations of the day, to perhaps show up the generosity of the Samaritan through the disbelief of the servants and/or the innkeeper's family.

APPENDIX

Administration on Aging, Office of Human Development, Department of Health, Education and Welfare, Washington, D.C., 20201

American Association of Occupational Therapy, 6000 Executive Blvd., Rockville, Maryland, 20852

American Association of Retired Persons, 215 Long Beach Blvd., Long Beach, California, 90801

American Dance Therapy Association, Inc., 2000 Century Plaza, Suite 230, Columbia, Maryland, 21044

American Psychological Association, Division of Adult Development and Aging, 1200 17th Street N.W., Washington, D.C., 20036

American Theatre Association, Senior Adult Theatre Program, 1000 Vermont Avenue, Washington, D.C., 20005

Ethel Percy Andrus Gerontology Center, University of California, Los Angeles, California, 90007

Expansion Arts Program, National Endowment for the Arts, Washington, D.C., 20506

Gerontological Society, One Dupont Circle, Washington, D.C., 20036

Gray Panthers, 3700 Chestnut St., Philadelphia, Pennsylvania, 19104

Institute of Gerontology, Lila Green, Program Coordinator in the Arts, University of Michigan, 520 East Liberty, Ann Arbor, Michigan, 48109

National Association of Activity Professionals, PO Box 274, Park Ridge, IL. 60068.

National Association of Social Workers, Suite 600, 1425 H Street N.W., Washington, D.C., 20005

National Center on the Arts and Aging, National Council on the Aging, Inc., 600 Maryland Avenue S.W., West Wing 100, Washington. D.C., 20024

National Committee on Art Education for the Elderly, Albert Beck, Executive Director, 520-5 Culver-Stockton College, Canton, Missouri, 63435

National Therapeutic Recreation Society, 1601 North Kent Street, Arlington, Virginia, 22209

New England Consortium for Gerontology, 25 Garrison Avenue, Durham, New Hampshire, 03824

Western Gerontological Society, 1095 Market Street, San Francisco, California, 94103

STORIES FOR DRAMATIZATION

(The numbers in ( ) at the end of each annotation correspond to the sources on the reference page.)

Androcles and the Lion. Androcles a runaway slave befriends a wounded lion who later refuses to eat him when they meet in the Roman arena. (1)

As We Are Now. This novel in journal style recounts the experiences of Caroline Spencer's day in a small rural nursing home. It chronicles her relation to the hypocrisy of the owner, the loss of privacy and the lack of sensory stimulation. Visits from a minister and a farmer's wife lighten her days, but her continual struggle to overcome isolation and hold on to reality give the book its poignancy and insights into institutional living. (16)

Baucis and Philemon. Baucis and Philemon, a loving peasant couple, welcome two strangers into their poor hut after others have refused hospitality. The strangers, actually gods, grant the wishes of the couple for their life on this earth and hereafter. (12)

Beautiful Blue Danube. While counting the laundry the wife of Johann Strauss notices notes written on the cuff of a shirt. As she hummed the tune, she was entranced, but unwittingly allowed the shirt to go to the laundress.
Once retrieved, the shirt bore the opening strains of the Blue Danube Waltz. (21)

The Cop and the Anthem. Soapy, a charming hobo, tries in vain to be arrested so he can spend the winter comfortably in jail. The story ends with a typical O. Henry surprise. (17)

Eagle, Wildcat and Sow. The wildcat plants the seeds of mutual distrust in the ears of the sow and eagle but ultimately fails to disrupt their friendship. (1)

A Family. An 85 year old grandfather suffers from advice and dependence on his family. (5)

First Friction Match. A French chemist saves the lives of explorers Lewis and Clark who have been captured by the Indians by magically igniting a pile of brush. The magic was the first friction match, the inventor was Jean Saugrain. (21)

The First Sundae. When ice cream sodas were outlawed on Sunday in Evanston, Illinois in 1874, an enterprising druggist sold ice cream without soda, calling them Sundaes. (21)

The Good Samaritan. The story of the Samaritan who rescues a stranger after he has been robbed and left to die along the road from Jericho to Jerusalem. (12)

Julie Romain. The story of a 69 year old actress who still feels 20. Each evening her servants enact for her a romantic scene in the garden. (5)

Julius Caesar. A ruthless pirate once captured a boy of ten and held him for ransom. For five days the boy's unearthly moaning strained the pirates' nerves. When finally released the boy vowed vengeance. Many years later, the boy, then Emperor of Rome, ordered the capture and death of the pirate. The boy was Julius Caesar. (21)

Lamb to the Slaughter. This story of Mary Maloney, who commits the "perfect crime," was adapted for the Alfred Hitchcock series on television. The reader sympathizes with Mary's situation and takes pleasure in the clever way in which she eludes detection. (4)

Landladies. After being bawled out by his landlady for making too much noise and having a woman in his room, Simple destroys all the signs that have been put up in the bathroom. The landlady locks him out of his room and will not allow him back until he pays his rent. (6)

The Man Who Made Trees Blossom. A Japanese tale about a couple who give away the gold coins dug up in the garden by their dog. Greedy neighbors borrow the dog but beat him to death when no riches are discovered on their land. The spirit of the dog grants magic powers to the old man which allows him to transform withered trees into blooming ones. Beauty is restored to the whole landscape of Japan. In recognition of the old man's deeds the prince rewards him and punishes the greedy couple. (12)

My Country Tis of Thee. Samuel Smith, Commissioned to write a national anthem for the United States after the Revolutionary War, used the tune of an old German hymn. Rejected at first because the music was the same as the British National Anthem, this song was accepted later as the national anthem of the United States. (21)

The Porcupine and the Snakes. A family of snakes offers a corner of their cave to a porcupine, only to be made strangers in their own house by the prickly stranger. (1)

A Pound of Kasha. Dorothy, the child of Polish immigrant parents, has difficulty communicating on her first trip alone to the grocery store. With some difficulty she discovered that "kasha" in Polish means "buckwheat groats" in English. (18)

Recall of Childhood. Blind and suffering from sciatica, tuberculosis and unable to use his right hand, Robert Louis Stevenson transcended his pain by recalling his childhood. Remembering the joys of the past he wrote the famous *Child's Garden of Verses.* (21)

Revelation: Diaries of Women. An excerpt of the diary of Florida Scott Maxwell, age 82, which describes events from her childhood and reveals her attitude about life, illness, beauty, womanhood and aging. (15)

The Shepherd Boy and the Wolf. The townspeople, fooled twice by the shepherd's faked cry of "Wolf" refuse to respond to the third call. (1)

Uncle Podger. Although Uncle Podger, an egocentric and cantankerous character, insists that he can hang a picture all by himself, he soon involves the whole family, complicating the process at each step. (2)

Valentine. The blind daughter of the jailor of a Roman prison befriends Valentine, a prisoner condemned because of his belief in Christianity. His farewell message to the girl in 207 AD became the first valentine. (2)

A Visit of Charity. A young girl visits two women in a nursing home in order to earn points for her Campfire badge. The girl is unprepared for the relationship of the two women and the ways they deal with reality. (24)

The Wolf and the Goat. A hungry wolf tried unsuccessfully to lure a goat down from a high cliff where he is browsing. (1)

POETRY FOR DRAMATIZATION

The number in ( ) at the end of each annotation correspond to the sources on the reference page.

America For Me. A traveler recalls and admires famous cities and countries of the world, but longs to return to his homeland, America. (13)

The Blind Man and the Elephant. A poetic version of the old Hindu tale of six blind men who dispute the nature of the elephant because each has explored a different part of the animal. (13)

The Chantey of Noah and the Ark. A ballad in which the townspeople scoff at Noah as he builds the ark, but are pleased when they see the animals come aboard. They believe Noah is starting a circus for their town. (7)

Clipper Days. An eighty year old man remembers his glorious days aboard a clipper ship and expresses his disgust with modern steam ships. (7)

Death of the Hired Man. A New England farmer and his wife exchange thoughts and feelings about Warren, a hired man who has come back to die on the farm. (20)

Dreams. An eight line poem attesting to the importance and necessity for dreams. (14)

The Enchanted Shirt. A king cuts off the heads of the doctors who fail to cure his illness, which is imaginary. He is finally advised to sleep for one night in the shirt of a happy man but alas, none can be found. Realizing the foolishness of his condition, the king cures himself. (19)

End of the War. Poems written by residents in the American Nursing Home in New York City about feelings and reactions to the end of World War II. (8)

Get Up and Bar the Door. After a heated argument over who should shut the cottage door, this stubborn couple agree that the next one who speaks must close the door. In the silence that ensues, two strangers enter and provide a reason for the old man to speak first. (20)

Hunting Song. This dramatic poem of a fox hunt will appeal to seniors who have hunted for sport. The contrast of the sly fox with the mad hounds provides strong visual images to accompany the galloping rhythm. (14)

I Never Told Anybody. Poems by residents of the American Nursing Home in New York City concerning secrets, fears, pranks never before shared. (8)

Johnny Sands. Tired of his life with a scolding wife, Johnny asks her help in drowning himself. She cheerfully agrees but is herself drowned instead. Humorous ballad. (7)

Little Lost Pup. A short poem depicting the joys of a lost pup and his new found master. (13)

Mother's Biscuits. This poem with strong sensory images can awaken childhood memories of mothers, kitchens and families. (14)

Mr. Zinnia. An itinerant handy man who appears each spring not only does the chores but shares bright zinnea seeds and tales of far off lands. (11)

On a Night of Snow. This poem is a dialogue between a concerned owner and her cat during a snow storm. The owner pleads with her cat to stay safe inside, but the cat demands that the door be opened. (14)

Oregon Winter. A short free verse poem which evokes the slower pace of the rainy winter months when at last the farmer can move unhurried while he whittles and dreams. (14)

Shanghaied. After swearing to give up the sea, a sailor is shanghaied onto yet another ship. (7)

Sound of Fire/Sound of Water. Two simple poems which appeal to the ear with strong imagery. (11)

Swift Things are Beautiful. This lyric poem contrasts swift things with slow ones. (14)

Unsatisfied Yearnings. A short poem which describes a dog's urgent need to be let out, and after he is out, his equally urgent desire to be let in. (14)

Woman With A Walk. A character study of a crippled woman who sells pencils in the park and her encounter with a little girl who is both intrigued and embarrassed to be seen with the lady. (11)

REFERENCES FOR DRAMATIZATION

1. *Aesop's Fables.* New York: Grosset and Dunlap. 1947

2. *Around and About.* Ed: Robert Bruce, Margaret Turker. London: English University Press, 1968.

3. Chilver, Peter. *Stories for Improvisation.* London: Batsford. 1969

4. Dahl, Roald. *Selected Stories of Roald Dahl.* New York: Modern Library. 1968

5. De Maupassant, Guy. *The Complete Short Stories of Guy De Maupassant.* New York, Garden City: Hanover House. 1955

6. Hughes, Langston. *The Best of Simple.* New York: Hill and Wang. 1961

7. Kemp, Harry. *Chanteys and Ballads.* New York: Brentanos. 1920

8. Koch, Kenneth. *I Never Told Anybody.* New York: Random House. 1977

9. Lester, Julius. *Black Folk Tales.* New York: Richard Barton. 1969

10. *Noodles, Nitwits, and Numbskulls.* Ed: Maria Leach. New York: Dell Pub. 1979

11. O'Neil, Mary. *People I'd Like to Keep.* Garden City, N.Y.: Doubleday and Co. N.D.

12. Payne, Philip. *Legend and Drama I.* London: Ginn and Co. Ltd. 1978

13. *The Poet's Craft.* Ed: Helen F. Daringer and Anne T. Eaton. New York: Granger Index Reprint Series. 1972

14. *Reflections on a Watermelon Pickle.* Ed: Stephen Dunning, Edward Leuders, Hugh Smith. Glenview, IL: Scott, Foresman and Co. 1966

15. *Revelations: Diaries of Women.* Ed: Mary Jane Moffatt and Charlotte Painter. New York: Vintage Books. 1975

16. Sarten, May. *As We Are Now.* New York: W.W. Norton. 1973

17. *Short Story Masterpieces.* Ed: Robert Penn Warren and Albert Erskine. New York: Dell Publishing Co. 1954

18. *Stories for Jewish Juniors.* Ed: Doris Gold. New York: Jonathan David. 1968

19. *Stories to Dramatize.* Ed: Winifred Ward. New Orleans, La: Anchorage Press. 1952, 1981

20. *Story Poems, An Anthology of Narrative Verse, 2nd Ed.* Ed: Louis Untermeyer. New York: Pocket Library. 1960

21. *This is the Story.* Morton Publishing Co. 1949

22. Thurber, James. *The Thurber Carnival.* New York: Harper Bros. N.D.

23. *Touchstones.* Ed: M.G. Benton and P. Benton. London: English University Press. N.D.

24. Welty, Eudora. *A Curtain of Green.* Garden City, N.Y.: Doubleday and Co. 1941

BIBLIOGRAPHY ON AGING AND DRAMA

BOOKS, ARTICLES, PAMPHLETS

Artists and the Aging, A Project Handbook. Ed.; COMPAS and St. Paul Ramsey Arts and Science Council. 1976. Washington, D.C.: National Council on the Aging, Inc.

Arts and the Aging: An Agenda for Action. Ed. Jacqueline T. Sunderland and Traylor Smith. Washington, D.C.: National Council on the Aging, Inc.

"The Arts and Aging: Forging a New Link." *Aging International,* Winter 1976. Available from: International Federation on Aging, 1009 K Street N.W., Washington, D.C. 20049.

Ball, W. L. The Meaning of Therapeutic Recreation. *Therapeutic Recreation Journal,* Vol. IV, No. 1, 1970.

Bennett, Ruth and Gurland, Barry. *The Acting Out Elderly.* New York: Haworth Press. 1981.

Berger, L. and Berger, M. A. Holistic Approach to the Psychogeriatric Patient. *International Journal of Group Psychotherapy.* Vol. 23, 1973.

Burger, Isabel. *Creative Drama for Senior Adults.* Wilton, Conn.: Morehouse Barlow Co. 1980.

Butler, Robert N. "The Life Review: An Interpretation of Reminiscence in the Aged." *Middle Age and Aging,* edited by Bernice L. Neugarten. Chicago: Chicago University Press, 1968.

Butler, R. and Lewis, M. *Aging and Mental Health.* St. Louis, Missouri: C. V. Mosby, 1977.

Caprow-Lindner, Erna, Harpaz, Leah and Samberg, Sonya. *Therapeutic Dance Movement: Expressive Activities for Older Adults.* New York: Human Sciences Press. 1979.

Cornish, Roger. "Senior Adult Theatre: The State of the Art and a Call for Research." *Theatre News,* May 1978.

Cornish, Roger and Orlock, John. *Short Plays for the Long Living.* Ed. Roger Cornish. Boston: Baker Plays, 1976.

Cranston, Jerneral. *Dramatic Imagination.* Interface California Corp. 1975.

Davis, Barbara. *Assessing the Impact of Creative Drama Training on Older Adults.* Unpublished PhD dissertation. The Pennsylvania State University. 1980.

Education: An Arts/Aging Answer. Ed. Jacqueline T. Sunderland and Traylor & Smith. Washington, D.C.: National Council on the Aging, Inc.

Etzkorn, Peter. "Arts & the Aging, Time for a Public Policy." *Perspective on Aging.* Washington, D.C.: National Council on the Aging, Inc.

Feil, Naomi. *Validation/Fantasy Therapy.* Cleveland, Ohio: Edward Feil Productions, 4614 Prospect Avenue. 1981.

———. "Group Therapy in a Home for the Aged." *The Gerontologist* 7 (3) Part 1 (September 1967).

Gray, Paula. *Dramatics for the Elderly.* New York: Columbia Teachers College Press. 1974.

Harbin, Shirley. *Dramatic Activities for the Elderly.* unpublished handbook. University of Michigan Institute of Gerontology. 1976.

Helm, J. B. and Gill, K. I. "An Essential Resource for the Aging, Dance Therapy." *Dance Research Journal of C.O.R.D.* Vol. III, No. 1, Fall-Winter 1974-5.

Hodgson, John and Richards, Ernest. *Improvisation.* New York: Grove Press. 1974.

Hoffman, Donald. *Pursuit of Arts Activities with Older Americans: An Administrative and Programmatic Handbook.* Washington, D.C.: National Council on the Aging, Inc.

————. "Stimulating the Elderly to Explore the Arts." *Art Education*, April 1977, Vol. 30. No. 4 (Special Issue).

Hoffman, Donald and Evelyn Masen. "The Relationship of Arts and Leisure to Elderly Person: An Annotated Bibliography." *Art Education*, April 1977, Vol. 30 No. 4 (Special Issue).

Humphrey, F. "Therapeutic Recreation and the 70's: Challenge or Progress." *Therapeutic Recreation Journal*. Vol. III. No. 8, 1970.

Jenkins, Sara. Past Present: *Recording Life Stories of Older People*. Washington, D.C.: National Council on the Aging, Inc.

Jennings, Sue. *Remedial Drama*. New York: Theatre Arts Books. 1978.

Kaminsky, Marc. *What's Inside You It Shines Out of You*. New York: Horizon Press.

Kartman, Lauraine L. "The Power of Music in a Nursing Home." *Activities, Adaptation & Aging*. Vol. 1, No. 1, Fall, 1980.

Keith, Pat M. "Life Changes, Leisure Activities and Well-Being Among Very Old Men and Women." *Activities, Adaptation & Aging*. Vol. 1, No. 1, Fall, 1980.

Klein, W. E., LeShaw, E. and Furman, S. *Promoting Mental Health of Older People Through Group Methods: A Practical Guide*. New York: Mental Health Materials Center. 1965.

Koch, Kenneth. *I Never Told Anybody: Teaching Poetry Writing in a Nursing Home*. New York: Random House. 1977.

Kubie, Susan and Landeau, Gertrude. *Group Work with the Aged*. New York: International University Press. 1969.

"Leisure & Aging: New Perspectives." *Leisure Today*. October 1977 (Special Issue).

Lerner, Arthur. *Poetry in the Therapeutic Experience*. New York: Pergamon Press. 1978.

Merrill, T. *Activities for the Aged and Infirm: A Handbook for the Untrained Worker*. Springfield, Il: Charles C. Thomas (5th Ed.) 1971.

Michaels, Claire. *Geridrama Manual*. (Unpublished Manual) 37-54 834d St.. Jackson Heights, New York.

Mosey, A. C. *Activities Therapy*. New York: Raven Press Pub. 1973.

Myerhoff, Barbara. *Number Our Days*. New York: Simon & Schuster. 1978.

Myerhoff, Barbara G. and Tufte, Virginia. "Life History as Integration: Personal Myth and Aging." *The Gerontologist*, 1975.

Perspectives: A Handbook in Drama and Theatre By, With and For Handicapped Individuals. Ed. Ann M. Shaw, Wendy Perks, C. J. Stevens. Washington, D.C.: American Theatre Association. 1981.

Polsky, Milton. *Let's Improvise*. Englewood Cliffs, N.J.: Prentice Hall. 1980.

————. "The Brookdale Drama Project," unpublished mimeographed report, Hunter College, 1976.

Reichenfeld, H. et al. "Evaluating the Effect of Activity Programs on a Geriatric Ward." *The Gerontologist*, Vol. 13. Summer 1972. p. 305-310.

Sarton, May. *As We Are Now*. New York: W. W. Norton. 1973.

————. *Kinds of Love*. New York: W. W. Norton. 1970.

Senior Adult Theatre: *The American Theatre Association Handbook*. Ed. Roger Cornish and Robert Kase. University Park. Pennsylvania: Pennsylvania State University Press. 1981.

Spolin, Viola. *Improvisation for the Theatre*. Evanston, Illinois: Northwestern University Press. 1963.

Sunderland, Jacqueline. "Art's Aglow with Rekindled Interest." *Perspectives on Aging*. Washington, D.C.: National Council on the Aging. Inc.

————. "National Center on Arts and the Aging: A Resource for Arts Educators." *Art Education*, April, 1977, Vol. 30, No. 4 (Special Issue).

————. *Older Americans and the Arts: A Human Equation*. Washington, D.C.: National Council on the Aging. Inc.

Timberman, Sandra. "Lifetime Learning and the Arts—A New Priority." *Art Education*. April 1977, Vol. 30, No. 4 (Special Issue).

Wagner, Betty Jane. *Dorothy Heathcote: Drama as a Learning Medium*. Washington, D.C.: National Education Association. 1976.

Way, Brian. *Development Through Drama*. New York: Humanities Press. 1967.

Wethered, A. G. *Movement and Drama in Therapy*. Boston: Plays, Inc. 1973.

PERIODICALS

Activities, Adaptation & Aging (Quarterly), Haworth Press, Inc., 28 East 22 St., New York 10010.

Adult Leadership (Monthly), Adult Education Association of the United States, 810 - 18th St. N.W., Washington, D.C. 20006.

Aging (Monthly), Administration on Aging, U. S. Department of Health, Education and Welfare, U. S. Printing Office, Washington, D.C. 20402.

American Journal of Occupational Therapy (Monthly), American Occupational Therapy Association, 6000 Executive Blvd., Rockville, Md. 10852.

CD News. Ed. Naida Weisburg, P.O. Box 2335, Providence, R.I. 02906.

CTTA Senior Adult Bulletin. Ed. Pat Whitton, Trolley Place, Connecticut.

Current Literature on Aging (Quarterly), National Council on the Aging, Inc., 600 Maryland Ave., S.W., West Wing 100, Washington, D.C. 20024.

The Gerontologist (Monthly), Lancet Publications, 4015 W. 65th St., Minneapolis, Minn. 55434.

Journal of Leisurability, Leisurability Publications, Box 281, Ottawa, Ontario, Canada KIN 8V2.

Modern Maturity (Semi-monthly), American Association of Retired Persons, 215 Long Beach, Cal. 90801.

Senior Adult Theatre Information Network (Quarterly), American Theatre Association, 1000 Vermont Ave., N.W., Washington, D.C. 20005.

Therapeutic Recreation Journal (Quarterly), National Therapeutic Recreation Society, 1601 N. Kent St., Arlington, Va. 22209.

DIRECTORY OF ACTIVITIES
AND SESSION PLANS

Activities and session plans are arranged, under each heading, beginning with the simpler ones and progressing to the more complex ones.

INDEX

T - #0551 - 101024 - C0 - 212/152/11 - PB - 9780789060372 - Gloss Lamination